# POCKET REFERENCE

## FOR THE
## EMT-B AND FIRST RESPONDER

**Bob Elling, MPA, REMT-P**

Prentice
Hall

Upper Saddle River, NJ 07458

Brady's Pocket Reference for the EMT-B and First Responder was designed to provide you, the EMT-B or First Responder, with a handy, pocket-size guide to which you can quickly refer.

*Dedicated to my wife Kirsten and my daughters Laura and Caitlin. May you always maintain humility as your accomplishments meet the stars.*

© 2003 by Pearson Education, Inc.

Upper Saddle River, NJ 07458

Printed in the United States of America

10  9  8  7  6  5

ISBN 0-13-098167-2

## ABOUT THE AUTHOR:

Bob Elling, MPA, REMT-P, is a Professor of Management for the American College of Prehospital Medicine, a faculty member for Hudson Valley Community College Institute of Prehospital Emergency Medicine, and a paramedic with the Town of Colonie EMS Department. Bob has served as a paramedic and Lieutenant for NYC*EMS, Associate Director of the New York State EMS Program, and Education Coordinator for "PULSE: Emergency Medical Update."

Special thanks go to Deborah Parks for her skillful editing of this manual.

It is the intent of the authors and publisher that this textbook be used as part of a formal EMT-Basic education program taught by qualified instructors and supervised by a licensed physician. The procedures described in this textbook are based upon consultation with EMT and medical authorities. The authors and publisher have taken care to make certain that these procedures reflect currently accepted clinical practice; however, they cannot be considered absolute recommendations.

The material in this textbook contains the most current information available at the time of publication. However, federal, state, and local guidelines concerning clinical practices, including without limitation, those governing infection control and universal precautions, change rapidly. The reader should note, therefore, that the new regulations may require changes in some procedures.

It is the responsibility of the reader to familiarize himself or herself with the policies and procedures set by federal, state, and local agencies as well as the institution or agency where the reader is employed. The authors and the publisher of this textbook and the supplements written to accompany it disclaim any liability, loss, or risk resulting directly or indirectly from the suggested procedures and theory, from any undetected errors, or from the reader's misunderstanding of the text. It is the reader's responsibility to stay informed of any new changes or recommendations made by any federal, state, and local agency as well as by his or her employing institution or agency.

# Contents

## Vital Signs and Patient Assessment

# Contents

## Airway Management and Breathing Skills

## Assessment Skills

# Contents

# Contents

# Contents

## Pediatric Patients

## Pregnancy and Birth

## Poisons

# Contents

# Contents

# Contents

I would like to thank Dr. Edward T. Dickinson and Daniel Limmer for their review of the second edition of this pocket reference. They offered significant contributions to the improvement of this guide, and I greatly appreciate their assistance.

**Edward T. Dickinson, MD, NREMT-P, FACEP**
Assistant Professor
Department of Emergency Medicine
School of Medicine
University of Pennsylvania
Philadelphia, Pennsylvania

**Daniel Limmer, EMT-P**
Faculty Member
Emergency Health Services
The George Washington University
Washington, D.C.

## ➤ NORMAL RESPIRATORY RATES (BREATHS PER MINUTE, AT REST)

| | |
|---|---|
| Adult | 12–20 |
| Adolescent (11–14) | 12–20 |
| School age (6–10) | 16–30 |
| Preschooler (3–5) | 20–30 |
| Toddler (1–3) | 20–30 |
| Infant (6–12 months) | 20–30 |
| Infant (0–5 months) | 25–40 |
| Newborn: | 30–50 |

## ➤ NORMAL RESPIRATORY RHYTHM

Regular.

## ➤ NORMAL RESPIRATORY QUALITY

Breath sounds are present and equal.
Chest expansion is adequate and equal.
Breathing takes minimum effort.

## ➤ NORMAL RESPIRATORY DEPTH

Adequate.

## ➤ RESPIRATORY SOUNDS/POSSIBLE CAUSES

*Snoring*—airway partially blocked.
*Wheezing*—asthma, anaphylaxis.
*Gurgling*—fluids in the airway.
*Crowing*—croup.

### ➤ RESPIRATORY IRREGULARITIES

*Breath sounds*—diminished, unequal, absent.
*Chest expansion*—inadequate or unequal.
*Effort of breathing*—labored, increased respiratory
  effort, accessory muscle use (may be pronounced
  in infants/children and involve nasal flaring, seesaw
  breathing, grunting, and retractions between ribs
  and above clavicles and sternum).

### ➤ NORMAL PULSE RATES (BEATS PER MINUTE, AT REST)

| | |
|---|---|
| Adult | 60–100 |
| Adolescent (11–14) | 60–105 |
| School age (6–10) | 70–110 |
| Preschooler (3–5) | 80–120 |
| Toddler (1–3) | 80–120 |
| Infant (6–12 months) | 80–140 |
| Infant (0–5 months) | 90–140 |
| Newborn: | 120–160 |

### ➤ PULSE IRREGULARITIES/POSSIBLE CAUSES

*Rapid, regular, and full*—exertion, fright, drugs, high
  blood pressure, first-stage blood loss.
*Rapid, regular, and thready*—shock, later stages of
  blood loss.
*Slow*—head injury, drugs, some poisons, some heart
  problems, hypoxia in children, well-conditioned
  athletes, hypothermia.
*No pulse*—cardiac arrest.

### ➤ NORMAL BLOOD PRESSURE

|  | **Systolic** | **Diastolic** |
|---|---|---|
| Adults | 90–150 | 60–90 |
| Infants/Children | 80 + 2 × age (years) | 2/3 systolic |
|   Adolescent | 88–140 | (average 59) |
|   School age | 80–122 | (average 57) |
|   Preschooler | 78–116 | (average 55) |

### ➤ BLOOD PRESSURE IRREGULARITIES/POSSIBLE CAUSES

*High blood pressure*—medical condition, exertion, fright, stress, emotional distress, excitement.

*Low blood pressure*—athlete or other person with normally low blood pressure, blood loss, late sign of shock.

### ➤ SKIN COLOR

*Pink*—normal in light-skinned patients; normal at inner eyelids, lips, and nailbeds of dark-skinned patients.

*Pale*—constricted blood vessels possibly resulting from blood loss, shock, hypotension, or emotional distress.

*Cyanotic*—lack of oxygen resulting from inadequate breathing or heart function.

*Flushed*—heat exposure, high blood pressure, emotional excitement.

*Jaundiced (yellow)*—abnormalities of the liver.

*Mottling*—occasionally in patients in shock.

## ➤ SKIN TEMPERATURE AND CONDITION

*Cool, clammy*—sign of shock.
*Cold, moist*—body is losing heat.
*Cold, dry*—exposure to cold.
*Hot, dry*—high fever, heat exposure.
*Hot, moist*—high fever, heat exposure.
*"Goose pimples" with shivering, chattering teeth, blue lips, and pale skin*—chills, exposure to cold, communicable disease, pain, fever.

## ➤ PUPIL IRREGULARITIES/POSSIBLE CAUSES

*Dilated*—fright, blood loss, drugs (e.g., Atropine), treatment with eye drops.
*Constricted*—drugs (narcotics), treatment with eye drops.
*Unequal*—stroke, head injury, eye injury, artificial eye.
*Lack of reactivity*—drugs, lack of oxygen to brain.

> **PUPIL GAUGE**

| | |
|---|---|
| • | 2 mm |
| ● | 3 mm |
| ● | 4 mm |
| ● | 5 mm |
| ● | 6 mm |
| ● | 7 mm |
| ● | 8 mm |
| ● | 9 mm |

➤ **FLOW CHARTS**

*Scene Size-up*

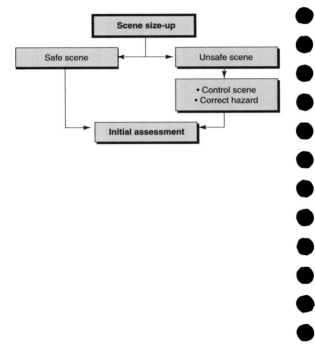

*Trauma Patient Assessment*

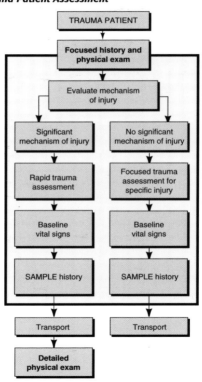

***Medical Patient Assessment***

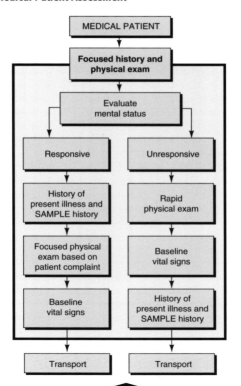

## ➤ SCALES, ACRONYMS, AND MNEMONICS

### Mental Status: AVPU

*A* — Alert. Awake and oriented.
*V* — Verbal. Responds to verbal stimulus.
*P* — Painful. Responds to painful stimulus.
*U* — Unresponsive. Does not respond to any stimulus.

| Glasgow Coma Scale | | |
|---|---|---|
| *Eye Opening* | Spontaneous | 4 |
| | To Voice | 3 |
| | To Pain | 2 |
| | None | 1 |
| *Verbal Responses* | Oriented | 5 |
| | Inappropriate Words | 4 |
| | Incomprehensible | 3 |
| | Sounds | 2 |
| | None | 1 |
| *Motor Response* | Obeys Commands | 6 |
| | Localizes Pain | 5 |
| | Withdraw (pain) | 4 |
| | Flexion (pain) | 3 |
| | Extension (pain) | 2 |
| | None | 1 |
| Glasgow Coma Scale Total | | |

**✱NOTE:** *During the initial assessment, AVPU is used for the quick neurological exam. During the focused physical exam, the Glasgow Coma Scale (GCS) may be used per local protocols.*

### OPQRST Questions

*O* — Onset. How did it start? What were you doing?

*P* — Provokes. Does anything make it better or worse?

*Q* — Quality. Can you describe it for me?

*R* — Radiation. Where exactly is the pain? Does it seem to spread anywhere, or does it stay right there?

*S* — Severity. Are you uncomfortable? How bad is the pain on a scale of 1 to 10?

*T* — Time. When did the pain start? Has it changed at all since it started?

### SAMPLE History

*S* — Signs/symptoms. Have you had any other symptoms?

*A* — Allergies. Are you allergic to anything?

*M* — Medications. What medicines do you take? What do you take those for?

*P* — Pertinent past history. Do you have any other medical problems? Have you ever had this kind of problem before? Who is your doctor?

*L* — Last oral intake. When was the last time you ate or drank anything? What did you eat or drink?

*E* — Events leading to the illness. How have you felt today? Anything out of the ordinary?

### DCAP-BTLS

*D* — Deformities.
*C* — Contusions.
*A* — Abrasions.
*P* — Punctures/penetrations.
*B* — Burns.
*T* — Tenderness.
*L* — Lacerations.
*S* — Swelling.

### High-Priority Conditions

- Poor general impression.
- Unresponsive.
- Responsive, but not following commands.
- Difficulty breathing.
- Shock.
- Complicated childbirth.
- Chest pain with systolic blood pressure less than 100.
- Uncontrolled bleeding.
- Severe pain anywhere.

### Significant Mechanisms of Injury (MOI)

- Ejection from vehicle.
- Death in same passenger compartment.
- Falls of more than 15 feet or three times the patient's height.
- Roll-over of vehicle.
- High-speed vehicle collision.
- Vehicle-pedestrian collision.
- Motorcycle crash.
- Unresponsiveness or altered mental status.
- Penetrations of the head, chest, or abdomen.

## ➤ 1—JAW-THRUST MANEUVER

- Take BSI precautions.
- Carefully keep the patient's head, neck, and spine aligned. Move the patient as a unit as you place him or her in a supine position.
- Then kneel approximately 18 inches above the head of the supine patient.
- Reach forward and gently place one hand on each side of patient's lower jaw. Run your fingers along jaw until you just pass the angle of the jaw.
- Stabilize the patient's head with your palms and forearms.
- Using your index fingers, push the angles of patient's lower jaw forward.
- To keep the mouth open, use an oropharyngeal airway on a patient with no gag reflex.
- Do not tilt or rotate the patient's head.

**NOTE:** *Remember the purpose of jaw-thrust maneuver is to open the airway without moving the head or neck from a neutral position.*

### ➤ 2—HEAD-TILT/CHIN-LIFT MANEUVER

- Take BSI precautions.
- Once the patient is supine, place one hand on the forehead. Place the fingertips of your other hand under the bony area at the center of patient's lower jaw.
- Tilt the head by applying gentle pressure to patient's forehead.
- Use your fingertips to lift chin and to support lower jaw. Move jaw forward to a point where lower teeth are almost touching upper teeth. Do not compress soft tissues under lower jaw.
- Do not close the patient's mouth. It is best to insert an oropharyngeal airway if the patient has no gag reflex.

➤ **3—OROPHARYNGEAL SUCTIONING**

- Take BSI precautions.
- Position yourself at patient's head, and turn patient onto his or her side.
- A rigid tip (Yankauer) is preferred. While it does not need to be measured, never lose sight of the tip.
- Measure a flexible suction catheter (distance between patient's ear lobe and corner of mouth, or center of mouth to angle of jaw).
- Turn suction unit on. Attach the catheter and test for suction.
- Open and clear the patient's mouth.
- Place the rigid pharyngeal tip so that the convex (bulging-out) side is against roof of patient's mouth. Insert tip just to the base of the tongue. Do not push tip down into the throat or larynx.
- Apply suction only after the tip of the catheter or rigid tip is in place, suctioning on the way out, moving tip from side to side. Suction for no longer than 15 seconds. (As per U.S. Department of Transportation, suction toddlers for no longer than 10 seconds and infants for no longer than 5 seconds.)
- Hyperventilate the patient with 100 percent oxygen.

## ➤ 4—MOUTH-TO-MASK WITH OXYGEN

- Take BSI precautions.
- Connect one-way valve to mask.
- Connect oxygen to inlet on face mask. Oxygen should be run at 15 lpm.
- Kneel about 18 inches above the head of the supine patient.
- Open the airway (manually or with adjunct).
- Position mask on patient's face so that the apex is over bridge of nose and the base is between lower lip and prominence of chin.
- Establish and maintain a proper mask-to-face seal (jaw-thrust maneuver) by placing both thumbs on top sides of mask and with index, third, and fourth fingers of each hand grasp lower jaw on each side, between angle of jaw and ear lobe, to jut the jaw forward.
- Ventilate patient at proper volume and rate. If supplemental oxygen is available, administer 6 to 7 mL/kg (which is approximately 400 to 600 mL) over 1 to 2 seconds. If no supplemental oxygen is available, deliver 10 mL/kg (which is approximately 700 to 1,000 mL) over 2 seconds.*
- Remove your mouth from port to allow for passive exhalation.

*The abbreviated version of volume and rate is: 400–600 mL of 100% oxygen in 1–2 sec. OR 700–1,000 mL room air in 2 sec. It will be expressed in this manner in later skills.*

✱*NOTE: Do not delay mouth-to-mask ventilation if oxygen is not immediately available.*

### ➤ 5—OROPHARYNGEAL (ORAL) AIRWAY INSERTION

- Take BSI precautions.
- Select appropriate size airway.
- Measure airway (center of mouth to angle of jaw, or corner of mouth to tip of ear lobe).
- Insert airway without pushing tongue back into throat. Insert upside down and flip 180 degrees over tongue, or insert straight in with a tongue blade holding tongue forward.
- Remove oropharyngeal airway quickly if patient gags.

### ➤ 6—NASOPHARYNGEAL (NASAL) AIRWAY INSERTION

- Take BSI precautions.
- Select appropriate size airway (diameter of patient's little finger). An alternative method is to measure from patient's nostril to earlobe or to angle of jaw.
- Measure airway (nostril to ear lobe).
- Lubricate nasopharyngeal airway with water-soluble gel.
- Fully insert airway with bevel facing nasal septum.

## ➤ 7—TWO-RESCUER BVM VENTILATION

- Take BSI precautions.
- Open the medical patient's airway using head-tilt, chin-lift maneuver.
- Suction and insert an oropharyngeal airway.
- Select correct bag-valve-mask size (adult, child, or infant). A pop-off valve is not acceptable!
- Kneel approximately 18 inches above the head of the supine patient.
- Position mask on patient's face so that the apex is over bridge of nose and the base is between the lower lip and prominence of chin.
- Position thumbs over top half of mask, index and middle fingers over bottom half.
- Use ring and middle fingers to bring patient's jaw up to mask and maintain head-tilt, chin-lift. *Tilt the head back as if you were trying to stand patient on his or her head!*
- The second rescuer should connect bag to mask, if not already done. While you maintain mask seal, second rescuer should squeeze the bag with two hands until patient's chest rises (400–600 mL of 100% oxygen in 1–2 sec. OR 700–1,000 mL room air in 2 sec.).
- The second rescuer should release pressure on the bag and let the patient exhale passively. While this occurs, the oxygen reservoir is refilling.

**\*NOTE:** *This technique may be used for a trauma patient by combining a jaw-thrust maneuver with manual stabilization of the head and neck.*

### ➤ 8—PREPARING OXYGEN DELIVERY SYSTEM

- Select desired cylinder. Check label and hydrostat date.
- Place cylinder in an upright position and stand to one side.
- Remove plastic wrapper or cap protecting cylinder outlet.
- Keep plastic washer (some set-ups).
- Crack main valve for 1 second to clean it out.
- Select correct pressure regulator and flowmeter.
- Place cylinder valve gasket on regulator oxygen port.
- Make certain that pressure regulator is closed.
- Align pins, or thread by hand.
- Tighten T-screw for pin yoke.
- Tighten with a wrench for a threaded outlet.
- Attach tubing and delivery device.

#### Oxygen Cylinder Sizes

*D cylinder*—contains 350 liters.
*E cylinder*—contains 625 liters.
*M cylinder*—contains 3,000 liters.
*G cylinder*—contains 5,300 liters.
*H cylinder*—contains 6,900 liters.

### ➤ 9—OXYGEN ADMINISTRATION VIA NONREBREATHER

- Take BSI precautions.
- Assemble regulator onto tank.
- Open main valve on tank.
- Check for leaks.
- Check tank pressure.
- Attach nonrebreather mask.
- Adjust liter flow to 12 to 15 liters per minute.
- Pre-fill reservoir.
- Apply and adjust mask to patient's face, explaining need for oxygen.
- Secure tank during transport.

### ➤ 10—OXYGEN ADMINISTRATION VIA NASAL CANNULA

- Take BSI precautions.
- Assemble regulator onto tank.
- Open main valve on tank.
- Check for leaks.
- Check tank pressure.
- Attach nasal cannula to regulator.
- Place nasal prongs into the patient's nose, and adjust tubing for patient comfort.
- Adjust liter flow to 1–6 lpm.
- Secure tank during transport.

### ➤ 11—DISCONTINUING OXYGEN ADMINISTRATION

- Remove delivery device from patient.
- Turn off the liter flow rate.
- Close the main valve.
- Remove the delivery tubing.
- Bleed the flowmeter.
- Change the tank if volume is 200 psi or less.

## ➤ 12—INSERTION OF ESOPHAGEAL TRACHEAL COMBITUBE® (EMT-B SKILL)

- Take BSI precautions.
- Position yourself at the patient's head.
- Assemble equipment.
- Insert the device blindly, watching for two black rings used for measuring depth of insertion. The teeth or their bony cavities, if teeth are missing, should be positioned between these rings.
- Use the large syringe to inflate the pharyngeal cuff with 100 cc of air. On inflation, the device will seat itself in the posterior pharynx behind the hard palate.
- Use the smaller syringe to fill the distal cuff with 10 cc to 15 cc of air.
- Usually (90–95 percent of the time), the tube will have been placed in the esophagus. On this assumption, ventilate through the esophageal connector (the external tube that is the longer of the two and is marked #1). You must listen for the presence of breath sounds in the lungs and the absence of sounds from the epigastrium in order to be sure that the tube is, in fact, placed in the esophagus.
- If there is an absence of lung sounds and presence of sounds in the epigastrium, the tube has been placed in the trachea. In this case, change the ventilator to the shorter tracheal connector, which is marked #2.
- Listen again to be sure of proper placement of the tube.

## ➤ 13—INSERTION OF THE LARYNGEAL MASK AIRWAY (LMA) ® (OPTIONAL EMT-B SKILL)

- Ensure that AHA BLS airway maneuvers are being attempted while preparing equipment.
- Take BSI precautions.
- Select and assemble correct equipment:
  - An LMA® properly sized for patient.
  - BVM with reservoir.
  - 30 cc syringe.
  - Suction unit and rigid Yankauer tip.
  - Test cuff by inflation and deflation.
  - Water-based lubricant gel for mask tip.
  - Gloves, mask, and protective eyewear.
- Have another rescuer hyperoxygenate the patient with a BVM.
- Place LMA®.
  - Gently introduce into oropharynx, following curvature of tube.
  - Swing mask into place in a single circular movement, ensuring pressure is maintained against palate and posterior pharynx.
  - Inflate mask without holding the tube.
  - Oxygenate the patient with the BVM.
- Confirm LMA® placement.
  - Visually confirm chest rise.
  - Auscultate epigastrium for absence of breath sounds.
  - Auscultate lung fields for presence of bilateral breath sounds.
  - Monitor $EtCO_2$.

- Properly secure the LMA® with tape and a bite block.
- Reassess the patient.
  - Confirm placement after LMA® is secured.
  - Reassess the ventilations for adequacy and depth.
- Document the procedure for PCR, confirming placement of the LMA® and the number of attempts.

## ➤ 14—ET INTUBATION & MANAGEMENT (EMT-B SKILL)

- Take BSI precautions.
- Open airway manually.
- Elevate tongue and insert airway adjunct (oropharyngeal or nasopharyngeal airway).
- Ventilate patient immediately using a BVM device attached to high concentration oxygen at the proper rate and volume.
- Direct assistant to hyperoxygenate patient.
- Identify and select proper equipment for intubation.
- Check equipment (cuffs for leaks, laryngoscope batteries, and bulb for tightness).
- Position head properly.
- Insert laryngoscope blade with left hand while displacing tongue.
- Elevate mandible with laryngoscope and visualize the vocal cords.
- Insert the ET and advance it to proper depth (until cuff is past vocal cords).
- Inflate cuff to proper pressure (5 cc to 10 cc of air) and disconnect syringe.
- Continue to hold onto the ET until it is secured in place.
- Direct ventilation of the patient.
- Confirm proper placement by auscultation bilaterally and over epigastrium.*
- Secure the ET tube with a commercial tube restraint.

*Some medical directors also require the use of an esophageal intubation detector device, pulse oximeter, colormetric end-tidal $CO_2$ device, or capnography to confirm proper tube placement.*

### ➤ 15—VENTILATING THE INTUBATED PATIENT

- Take BSI precautions.
- Position yourself at the patient's head.
- Look at the graduations on side of tube (e.g., adult male, 22 cm at teeth).
- Hold the tube against the patient's teeth with two fingers.
- Attach BVM to oxygen regulator and ET tube.
- Ventilate at a minimum of once every 5 seconds while watching the chest rise.
- Pay close attention to what ventilations feel like. Report any change in resistance.
- With each defibrillation attempt, carefully remove the bag from the tube.
- Watch for any change in the patient's mental status. A patient who becomes more alert may need to be physically or chemically restrained (by the paramedics) to prevent him or her from pulling out the tube.

**\*NOTE:** *Be especially careful not to disturb the ET tube. If it is pushed in, it will most likely enter the right mainstem bronchus, preventing oxygen from entering patient's left lung. If it is pulled out, it can easily slip into esophagus and send all ventilations directly to stomach, denying the patient oxygen. This is a fatal complication if it goes unnoticed. The tube placement should be monitored using capnography.*

## ➤ 16—OROTRACHEAL SUCTIONING (EMT-B SKILL)

- Take BSI precautions.
- Position yourself at the patient's head.
- Hyperventilate the patient.
- Carefully check equipment.
- Don sterile gloves.
- Grasp catheter with sterile gloved hand, and connect it to the suction device.
- Stop ventilations, occlude suction, and insert catheter into ET tube.
- Catheter may be advanced as far as carina.
- Advance catheter to desired level, apply suction, and withdraw catheter with twisting motion, no more than 15 seconds for adults.
- Start ventilations, and rinse catheter in sterile solution.
- Suction again as needed.

*✱NOTE: This is a sterile procedure throughout.*

### ➤ 17—INSERTION OF NASOGASTRIC TUBE (EMT-B SKILL)

- Take BSI precautions.
- Prepare and assemble the equipment.
- Oxygenate the patient.
- Measure tube from tip of nose, over ear, to below xiphoid process.
- Lubricate end of tube, and pass tube gently downward along nasal floor to stomach.
- To confirm correct placement, auscultate over epigastrium. Listen for bubbling while injecting 10 to 20 cc air into tube.
- Use suction to aspirate stomach contents.
- Secure tube in place.

## ➤ 18—USING THE PULSE OXIMETER

- Review the instruction manual for the specific unit you are using.
- Properly assemble finger-clip sensor and extension to pulse oximeter.
- Properly affix finger-clip sensor to index finger. (It may be necessary to quickly remove patient's fingernail polish.)
- Turn on pulse oximeter, and record heart and oxygen readings. Spot-check mode and extended mode (30 minutes).
- When done using oximeter, shut off the unit. After each use, disassemble and store wiring and accessories in pouch provided.
- Review operation of all display indicators, pulse amplitude, low battery, pulse search, oxygen saturation, and pulse rate.
- Review all controls (i.e., measure button, battery check button, printer on/off, printer paper advance).
- Change battery and paper printout if needed.

### ➤ 19—BLOOD PRESSURE BY AUSCULTATION

- Place stethoscope around your neck.
- Patient should be seated or lying down.
- If patient has not been injured, support his or her arm at heart level.
- Place cuff snugly around upper arm so that bottom of cuff is about 1 inch above crease of elbow.
- With your fingertips, palpate brachial artery at crease of elbow.
- Place the tips of stethoscope in your ears.
- Position the diaphragm of the stethoscope directly over the brachial pulse or over medial anterior elbow if no brachial pulse can be felt.
- Inflate cuff with bulb valve closed.
- Once you no longer hear brachial pulse, continue to inflate cuff until gauge reads 30 mm Hg higher than the point where pulse sound disappeared.
- Slowly release air from cuff by opening bulb valve, allowing pressure to fall smoothly at rate of approximately 10 mm per second.
- When you hear the first clicking or tapping sounds, note the reading on the gauge. This is the systolic pressure.
- Continue to deflate cuff and listen for point at which these distinctive sounds fade. When sounds turn to dull, muffled thuds, the reading on gauge is the diastolic pressure.
- After obtaining diastolic pressure, let cuff deflate rapidly.

### ➤ 20—BLOOD PRESSURE BY PALPATION

- Find radial pulse on the arm to which blood pressure cuff is applied.
- With bulb valve closed, inflate cuff to a point where you can no longer feel the radial pulse.
- Note this point on gauge, and continue to inflate cuff until gauge reads 30 mm Hg higher than point where pulse disappeared.
- Slowly deflate cuff, noting the reading at which the radial pulse returns. This reading is the systolic pressure.
- After obtaining systolic reading, let cuff deflate.

**NOTE*: You cannot determine diastolic reading by palpation.*

## ➤ 21—INITIAL ASSESSMENT

- Take BSI precautions.
- Form a general impression based on assessment of environment and patient's chief complaint and appearance.
- Assess mental status. Determine level of responsiveness using AVPU (alert, verbal, painful, unresponsive).
- Assess airway and breathing (assess, initiate appropriate oxygen therapy, assure adequate ventilation).
- Assess circulation (assess for and control major bleeding; assess pulse; assess skin color, temperature, and condition).
- Determine patient's treatment priority (high/low, C.U.P.S.), and make transport decision.

*NOTE: Apply manual stabilization on first contact with any patient who you suspect may have an injury to the spine.*

### ➤ 22—FOCUSED HISTORY AND PHYSICAL EXAM—RESPONSIVE MEDICAL PATIENT

- Take BSI precautions.
- Gather history of present illness from patient by asking OPQRST questions.
- Gather a SAMPLE history from patient.
- Conduct a focused physical exam (focusing on the area patient complains of).
- Obtain baseline vital signs.
- Perform interventions and contact on-line medical direction as needed.
- Transport (re-evaluate transport decision).

### ➤ 23—FOCUSED HISTORY AND PHYSICAL EXAM—UNRESPONSIVE MEDICAL PATIENT

- Take BSI precautions.
- Conduct a rapid physical exam, by assessing:
  - Head.
  - Neck.
  - Chest.
  - Abdomen.
  - Pelvis.
  - Extremities.
  - Posterior.
- Obtain baseline vital signs.
- Gather history of the present illness from bystanders or family by asking OPQRST questions.
- Gather a SAMPLE history from bystanders or family.
- Perform interventions (obtain medical direction as required locally). Reassess vital signs.
- Transport (re-evaluate transport decision).

### ➤ 24—FOCUSED HISTORY AND PHYSICAL EXAM— TRAUMA PATIENT, NO SIGNIFICANT MOI

- Take BSI precautions.
- Reconsider MOI.
- Determine patient's chief complaint.
- Conduct a focused physical exam (focusing on the area patient complains of plus areas of potential injury suggested by the MOI).
- Obtain baseline vital signs.
- Take a SAMPLE history.
- Perform interventions as needed.
- Transport.

### ➤ 25—FOCUSED HISTORY AND PHYSICAL EXAM— TRAUMA PATIENT, SIGNIFICANT MOI

- Take BSI precautions.
- Reconsider MOI.
- Continue manual stabilization of head and neck.
- Consider requesting ALS personnel.
- Reconsider your transport decision.
- Reassess mental status.
- Perform a rapid trauma assessment. After assessing head and neck, apply a cervical collar and continue to maintain manual stabilization.
- Obtain baseline vital signs.
- Take a SAMPLE history.
- Perform a detailed physical exam either on scene, if there is time, or en route to the hospital.
- Perform ongoing assessment, including vital signs.
- Transport.

## ➤ 26—RAPID TRAUMA ASSESSMENT

- Take BSI precautions.
- Assess head: DCAP-BTLS + crepitation.
- Assess neck: DCAP-BTLS + jugular vein distention (JVD) and crepitation.
- Assess chest: DCAP-BTLS + paradoxical motion, crepitation, breath sounds.
- Assess abdomen: DCAP-BTLS + firmness, softness, distention.
- Assess pelvis: DCAP-BTLS + pain, tenderness, motion.
- Assess extremities: DCAP-BTLS + distal pulse, motor function, and sensation.
- Assess posterior: DCAP-BTLS.

## ➤ 27—DETAILED PHYSICAL EXAM

- Take BSI precautions.
- Examine head: DCAP-BTLS + crepitation.
- Examine scalp and cranium: DCAP-BTLS + crepitation.
- Examine face: DCAP-BTLS.
- Examine ears: DCAP-BTLS + drainage.
- Examine eyes: DCAP-BTLS + discoloration, unequal pupils, foreign bodies, blood in anterior chamber.
- Examine nose: DCAP-BTLS + drainage, bleeding.
- Examine mouth: DCAP-BTLS + loose or broken teeth, objects that could cause obstruction, swelling or laceration of tongue, unusual breath odors, discoloration.
- Examine neck: DCAP-BTLS + jugular vein distention (JVD), crepitation.
- Examine chest: DCAP-BTLS + paradoxical motion, crepitation, breath sounds.
- Examine abdomen: DCAP-BTLS + firmness, softness, distention.
- Examine pelvis: DCAP-BTLS + pain, tenderness, motion.
- Examine extremities: DCAP-BTLS + distal pulse, motor function, sensation.
- Examine posterior: DCAP-BTLS.
- Reassess vital signs.

## ➤ 28—ONGOING ASSESSMENT

- Take BSI precautions.
- Repeat initial assessment for life-threats:
  - Reassess mental status.
  - Maintain open airway.
  - Monitor breathing rate and quality.
  - Reassess pulse rate and quality.
  - Monitor skin color, temperature, and condition.
  - Reestablish patient treatment priorities.
- Reassess and record vital signs.
- Repeat focused assessment related to chief complaint or injuries.
- Check interventions.
  - Assure adequacy of oxygen delivery and ventilation support.
  - Assure management of bleeding.
  - Assure adequacy of interventions.

**\*NOTE:** *Repeat the ongoing assessment every 15 minutes for a stable patient, every 5 minutes for an unstable patient.*

## ➤ 29—APPLYING STANDARD THREE-LEAD ECG ELECTRODES

- Take BSI precautions.
- Turn on the ECG monitor.
- Plug in monitoring cables or leads.
- Attach monitoring cables to electrodes.
- Apply electrodes to patient's body. The most common initial configuration is lead II, which involves placing the negative lead on the right shoulder area of chest, the ground lead on the left shoulder of the chest, and the positive lead on the left lower chest.

**NOTE:* *In very hairy patients, it may be necessary to shave electrode attachment points on chest.*

### ➤ 30—APPLYING TWELVE-LEAD ECG ELECTRODES

- Take BSI precautions.
- Turn on the ECG monitor.
- Plug in monitoring cables or leads.
- Attach monitoring cables to electrodes.
  Apply electrodes to patient's body, using the following locations for each electrode.
  - *V1*—Fourth intercostal space at the right border of the sternum.
  - *V2*—Fourth intercostal space at left border of the sternum.
  - *V3*—Midway between locations V2 and V4.
  - *V4*—At the mid-clavicular line in the fifth intercostal space.
  - *V5*—At the anterior axillary line on the same horizontal as V4.
  - *V6*—At the mid-axillary line on the same horizontal level as V4 and V5.
  - *RA*—Anywhere on the right arm.
  - *LA*—Anywhere on the left arm.
  - *RL*—Anywhere on the right leg.
  - *LL*—Anywhere on the left leg.

### ➤ 31-SETTING UP AND RUNNING AN IV LINE

- Take BSI precautions.
- Inspect fluid bag for clarity, expiration date, and leaks. Remove outer wrapper and gently squeeze bag.
- Verify type of solution with ALS provider.
- Select proper administration set, uncoil tubing, and keep ends sterile.
- Connect an extension set, if using a mini-drip.
- Make sure flow regulator is closed by rolling stop-cock away from direction of fluid bag.
- Remove protective coverings from port of fluid bag and spiked end of tubing. Insert spiked end of tubing into fluid bag with a quick twist.
- Hold fluid bag higher than drip chamber. Squeeze drip chamber one or two times to start flow. Fill chamber marker line (one-third full).
- Open flow regulator, and allow fluid to flush all air from tubing. You may need to loosen cap at lower end to get fluid flowing. *Be very careful to maintain sterility and to replace cap.*

### ➤ 32—REPOSITIONING ADULT PATIENT FOR BLS

- Take BSI precautions.
- Straighten patient's legs and position arm closest to you above his or her head.
- Cradle patient's head and neck. Grasp under the distant armpit.
- Move patient as a unit onto his or her side.
- Move patient onto back and reposition the extended arm.

*NOTE: This maneuver is used to initiate airway evaluation, artificial ventilation, or CPR when rescuer must act alone. When trauma is suspected, a four-rescuer log roll is the preferred technique.*

### ➤ 33—ONE-RESCUER CPR—ADULT PATIENT

- Take BSI precautions.
- Establish unresponsiveness.
- Activate the EMS system and ensure delivery of the AED.
- Open airway (head-tilt/chin-lift or jaw thrust).
- Check breathing (look, listen, feel).
- Give 2 slow breaths* and watch chest rise. Allow for exhalation between breaths.
- Check carotid pulse and other signs of circulation. If breathing is absent but pulse is present, provide rescue breathing (1 breath every 5 seconds; 12 breaths per minute).
- If no pulse, give cycles of 15 chest compressions (at rate of 100 per minute) followed by 2 slow breaths.
- Upon arrival of the AED at the patient's side, take the following steps:
  - Place AED next to patient. Then turn on the power.
  - Attach electrodes (sternum and apex).
  - Clear victim, and press analyze button.
  - If AED advises to shock, assure all are clear and then deliver the shock.
  - After series of shocks (per local protocol), assess pulse and signs of circulation.
  - Continue CPR until ALS arrives, and prepare for transport.
- After four cycles of 15:2 (about 1 minute), check pulse and signs of circulation. If no pulse, continue 15:2 cycle beginning with chest compressions.

*(continued)*

*Ventilations should be done using a bag-valve-mask (400–600 mL of 100 % oxygen in 1–2 sec. OR 700–1,000 mL room air in 2 sec.).*

**NOTE:** *If patient is breathing or resumes effective breathing and no trauma is suspected, place in recovery position.*

### ➤ 34—TWO-RESCUER CPR—ADULT PATIENT

- Take BSI precautions.
- Establish unresponsiveness.
- Assure EMS system has been activated and that the AED is on the way.

#### Rescuer A:

- Open airway (head-tilt/chin-lift or jaw-thrust).
- Check breathing (look, listen, feel).
- Give 2 slow breaths* and watch chest rise. Allow for exhalation between breaths.
- Check carotid pulse and other signs of circulation.

#### Rescuer B:

- If no pulse and other signs of circulation, give cycles of 15 chest compressions (at a rate of 100 per minute) followed by 2 slow breaths* by Rescuer A.
- After 1 minute of rescue support, recheck pulse and signs of circulation.
- If no pulse, continue 15:2 cycles.

*Ventilation should be done using a bag-valve-mask (400–600 mL of 100% oxygen in 1–2 sec. OR 700–1,000 mL room air in 2 sec.).*

## ➤ 35—CHECKING THE AED

Check the AED for the following:
- Unit, cables, connectors for cleanliness.
- Supplies carried with AED.
- Power supply and its operation.
- Indicators on ECG display.
- ECG recorder operation.
- Charge display cycle with a simulator.
- Pacemaker feature, if applicable.
- File a written report on status of AED.

**✱*NOTE: This list is derived from* FDA Automated Defibrillator: Operator's Shift Checklist.*

### ➤ 36—MOVING WHILE PERFORMING CPR

- Take BSI precautions.
- Confirm effectiveness of CPR (ventilations and compressions).
- Place a long backboard under patient, interrupting for maximum of 7 seconds.
- Resume CPR, prepare to lift on signal.
- On signal, quickly transfer patient and spine board to litter.
- Move litter slowly so CPR can continue.
- Before moving downstairs, pause briefly at landing, continuing CPR.
- On signal, stop CPR and move quickly to next landing and resume CPR for maximum 30 seconds.
- Move safely down the stairs.
- Begin CPR again.

**✱NOTE:** *If the patient has an IV or ET tube, be extremely careful when moving him or her.*

### ➤ 37—USING THE THUMPER®

- Take BSI precautions.
- Assure CPR is in progress and effective.
- Attach Thumper® base plate to long backboard.
- Stop CPR to slide long backboard under patient.
- Restart CPR and attach shoulder straps to patient.
- Slide Thumper® piston plate into position on base plate (away from chest).
- Stop CPR and quickly pivot piston arm into place, measuring anterior/posterior and middle sternum placement.
- Slowly adjust depth of compression to appropriate diagram.
- Adjust ventilations.
- Turn off compressions temporarily for pulse checks and defibrillation.
- Upon termination of arrest or return of pulses, power down unit.

**✱**NOTE: *Always store with compression depth turned down to minimum setting.*

## ➤ 38—FBAO—CONSCIOUS ADULT

- Ask: "Are you choking?" "Can you speak?"
- If choking and can't speak, give abdominal thrusts (chest thrusts for pregnant or obese patient).
- Repeat thrusts until effective or patient becomes unconscious.

### ➤ 39—FBAO—ADULT BECOMES UNCONSCIOUS

- Take BSI precautions.
- Activate the EMS system.
- Perform a tongue-jaw lift followed by a finger sweep to remove object.
- Open airway and try to ventilate. If still obstructed, reposition head and try to ventilate again.
- Give up to 5 abdominal thrusts.
- Repeat last three steps until obstruction is cleared.

**\*NOTE:** *If patient is breathing or resumes effective breathing, place in recovery position.*

### ➤ 40—FBAO—UNCONSCIOUS ADULT

- Take BSI precautions.
- Establish unresponsiveness.
- Activate the EMS system.
- Open airway, and check breathing.
- Try to ventilate. If obstructed, reposition head and try to ventilate again.
- Give up to 5 abdominal thrusts.
- Perform a tongue-jaw lift followed by a finger sweep to remove object.
- Repeat last three steps until the obstruction is cleared. Continue steps of CPR, if cleared.

**\*NOTE:** *If patient is breathing or resumes effective breathing, place in recovery position.*

### ➤ 41—BLEEDING CONTROL/SHOCK MANAGEMENT

- Take BSI precautions.
- Apply direct pressure to wound.
- Elevate the extremity.
- Apply a dressing to wound.
- If wound continues to bleed, apply an additional dressing to wound.
- If wound continues to bleed, locate and apply pressure to appropriate arterial pressure point.
- Apply high-concentration oxygen.
- Properly position patient.
- Initiate steps to prevent heat loss from patient.
- Indicate need for immediate transport.

### ➤ 42—APPLICATION OF PASG

- Take BSI precautions.
- Assure patient meets local protocol for PASG.
- Check for contraindications (e.g., pulmonary edema or penetrating chest injury).
- Remove clothing and check for sharp objects.
- Quickly assess areas that will be under PASG.
- Position PASG with top of abdominal section at or below last set of ribs.
- Secure PASG around patient.
- Attach hoses.
- Check patient's blood pressure.
- Begin inflation sequence.
- Stop inflation sequence at 106 mm Hg or pop-off valves release.
- Operate PASG to maintain air pressure in device.
- Reassess patient's vital signs.

*WARNING: Do not actually inflate a PASG on a mock victim in class.*

**\*NOTE:** MAST (military antishock trousers) is another name for the PASG.*

### ➤ 43—IMMOBILIZATION: LONG BONE

- Take BSI precautions.
- Direct application of manual stabilization.
- Assess distal pulses, motor ability, and sensory response (PMS).
- Measure splint.
- Apply splint.
- Immobilize joints above and below injury.
- Secure entire injured extremity from distal to proximal direction.
- Immobilize hand/foot in functional position.
- Reassess distal PMS.

### ➤ 44—REALIGNING AN EXTREMITY

- Take BSI precautions.
- Assess distal pulses, motor ability, and sensory response (PMS).
- Rescuer A grasps distal extremity, while Rescuer B places one hand above and below injury site.
- Rescuer B supports injury site, while Rescuer A pulls gentle manual traction in direction of long axis of body. If resistance is felt or if it appears that bone ends will come through skin, stop realignment and splint extremity in position found.
- If no resistance is felt, maintain gentle traction until extremity is properly splinted.
- Reassess distal PMS.

### ➤ 45—IMMOBILIZATION: JOINT INJURY

- Take BSI precautions.
- Direct application of manual stabilization of injury.
- Assess distal pulses, motor ability, and sensory response (PMS).
- Select proper splinting device.
- Immobilize the site of injury and the bones above and below.
- Reassess distal PMS.

### ➤ 46—IMMOBILIZATION: TRACTION SPLINT

- Take BSI precautions.
- Direct manual stabilization of injured leg.
- Assess distal pulses, motor ability, and sensory response (PMS).
- Direct application of manual traction.
- Adjust and position splint at the injured leg.
- Apply proximal securing device (e.g., ischial strap).
- Apply distal securing device (e.g., ankle hitch).
- Apply mechanical traction.
- Position and secure support straps.
- Reassess distal PMS.
- Secure patient's torso and traction splint to long backboard for transport.

## ➤ 47—SPINAL IMMOBILIZATION: SUPINE PATIENT

- Take BSI precautions.
- Direct assistant to place head in neutral, in-line position and to maintain manual stabilization until the patient is completely immobilized.
- Assess distal pulses, motor ability, and sensory response (PMS).
- Apply a properly sized rigid extrication collar.
- Position immobilization device appropriately.
- Move patient onto device without compromising integrity of spine. Apply padding to voids between torso and board as needed.
- Immobilize patient's torso to device.
- Evaluate and pad behind patient's head as necessary.
- Pad and immobilize patient's head.
- Secure patient's arms and legs to board.
- Reassess distal PMS.

### ➤ 48—SPINAL IMMOBILIZATION: SEATED PATIENT

- Take BSI precautions.
- Direct assistant to manually stabilize head in neutral, in-line position.
- Assess distal pulses, motor ability, and sensory response (PMS).
- Apply a properly sized rigid extrication collar.
- Position immobilization device behind the patient.
- Secure device to the patient's torso.
- Evaluate and pad behind head as needed.
- Secure patient's head to device.
- Evaluate and adjust straps.
- Secure wrists and legs.
- Reassess distal PMS.
- Transfer patient to long backboard.

➤ **49—RAPID EXTRICATION**

### Step 1: Perform an initial assessment.

- *Rescuer A:* Maintain manual stabilization of patient's head and neck.
- *Rescuer B:* Conduct initial assessment of patient and determine need for rapid extrication based on patient status. Assess pulses, motor ability, and sensory response (PMS) in four extremities.

### Step 2: Apply a cervical collar.

- *Rescuer B:* Apply a properly sized cervical collar.
- *Rescuer A:* Continue to maintain manual stabilization before, during, and after application of collar.

### Step 3: Lift patient and position the long backboard.

- *Rescuer B:* Hold patient's armpit, and join hands with Rescuer C under patient's thighs.
- *Rescuer A:* Call for a lift, while maintaining manual stabilization.
- *Rescuers B:* Lift patient approximately 2 inches off seat with Rescuer C.
- *Bystander (or 4th Rescuer):* Insert long backboard under patient on seat.

### Step 4: Begin to position patient for extrication.

- *Rescuer B:* Reach across patient's chest and support by both armpits.
- *Rescuer A:* While maintaining manual stabilization, call for one-fourth turn, so patient is moved perpendicular to steering wheel, ready to exit car head first.

*(continued)*

- *Rescuer C:* Free patient's lower legs from any obstructions.
- *Rescuer B:* Begin to turn patient's back toward door until Rescuer A says "stop turn."
- *Rescuer A:* Turn patient. Call for "stop turn" just before being unable to hold patient's head anymore.
- *Rescuer C:* Begin to turn patient's back toward door, freeing legs, then sliding up to thighs until Rescuer A says "stop."

### Step 5: Complete another one-fourth turn.

- *Rescuer B:* Stop move and wait for Rescuer C. Then take over manual stabilization of head and neck from Rescuer A.
- *Rescuer A:* Maintain head/neck stabilization until Rescuer B takes over, allowing him or her to either exit car and work from outside or reach over seat from inside if there is room or if roof has been removed.
- *Rescuer C:* Move hands from thighs to patient's armpits. Then replace Rescuer B.
- *Rescuers A, B, and C:* Complete another one-fourth turn.

### Step 6: Lower patient onto the long backboard.

- *Rescuer B:* Lower patient onto long backboard.
- *Rescuer A:* Call for move to lower patient's torso into a supine position on the long backboard.
- *Rescuer C:* Lower patient onto long backboard.
- *Bystander (or 4th Rescuer):* Stabilize the board.

*(continued)*

### Step 7: Position patient on the backboard.

- *Rescuer B:* Slide patient as a unit.
- *Rescuer A:* Call for move to slide patient toward head end of backboard. Once in position, tell partners to "stop." Slide chest as a unit.
- *Rescuer C:* Slide pelvis as a unit until Rescuer A says "stop."
- *Bystander (or 4th Rescuer):* Stabilize head end of long backboard.

### Step 8: Secure patient to the backboard.

- Crew carefully straps patient's torso first, head last, and then moves backboard to stretcher.
- Reassess PMS.

## ➤ 50—RAPID TAKEDOWN OF STANDING PATIENT

### *Step 1: Rescuers get in position.*

- *Rescuer A:* Get in position behind patient and hold manual in-line stabilization of head and neck. Maintain manual stabilization until the patient is completely immobilized on a long backboard.
- *Rescuer B:* Get in position in front of patient. Explain procedure so patient does not move.

### *Step 2: Assess PMS and apply a cervical collar.*

- *Rescuer B:* Quickly assess pulses, motor ability, and sensory response (PMS) in all four extremities.
- *Rescuer B:* Apply a properly sized rigid extrication collar.

### *Step 3: Position the long backboard.*

- Position long backboard behind patient, being careful not to disturb manual stabilization in any way.
- Standing in front of patient to each side, reach under patient's armpit and grasp backboard handhold at level of arm pit or higher. Both rescuers must hold same level.
- Then place your other hand on patient's upper arm, securing patient to backboard by holding it on board.

*(continued)*

### Step 4: Slowly lower the patient.

- Slowly lower patient backwards, communicating with Rescuer A behind board so it is clear when the scapulae are beginning to rest on board. Remember to lift with your legs, bending at knees not at waist. Rescuer A gently allows the head to come back to board as shoulders come back.
- Once head is on board, it never is lifted off board again as Rescuer A kneels down at patient's head.
- Reassess PMS when the patient is finally down.

### ➤ 51—WATER RESCUE: POTENTIAL SPINE INJURY

- Take BSI precautions.
- Conduct an initial assessment.
- Splint head and neck with arms. (Lift the patient's arms over his or her head. Then splint head and neck between arms.)
- Roll patient over into supine position.
- Assess airway and breathing. (Note: If patient is not breathing, remove him or her from water on a backboard as soon as possible.)
- Provide manual stabilization of head/neck.
- Assess pulses, motor ability, and sensory response (PMS) in four extremities.
- Slide backboard under patient.
- Apply a properly sized rigid extrication collar.
- Tie down torso, then head/neck with straps.
- Float board to edge of the water.
- Remove patient from water with as much assistance as needed.
- Obtain baseline vital signs.
- Conduct focused history and physical exam.
- Reassess PMS in four extremities.
- Apply oxygen, and prepare to transport.

### ➤ 52—ONE-RESCUER ASSIST

- Place patient's arm around your neck.
- Grasp patient's hand in your hand.
- Place your other arm around the patient's waist.
- Help patient walk to safety, communicating with him or her about obstacles or uneven terrain.

### ➤ 53—TWO-RESCUER ASSIST

- Each rescuer stands at one side of the patient.
- Each places a patient's arm around his or her shoulder and grips the patient's hand.
- Both rescuers then help the patient walk to safety.

## ➤ 54—EXTREMITY CARRY

### *Rescuer A:*

- Place the patient on his or her back with knees flexed.
- Kneel at patient's head, and place your hands under patient's shoulders.

### *Rescuer B:*

- Kneel at the patient's feet and grasp his or her wrists.
- Lift patient forward, while Rescuer A slips arms under patient's armpits and grasps patient's wrists.
- Grasp patient's knees while facing patient, or turn and grasp patient's knees while facing away from patient.

### *Rescuers A and B:*

- Crouch, then stand at the same time.
- Move as a unit when carrying the patient.

### ➤ 55—DIRECT CARRY

- ***Rescuers A and B:*** Get in position along one side of patient. Rescuer A is at head-end; Rescuer B at foot-end.
- ***Rescuer A:*** Cradle patient's head and neck by sliding one arm under patient's neck to grasp shoulder.
- ***Rescuer B:*** Slide hand under patient's hip and lift slightly.
- ***Rescuer A:*** Slide your other arm under patient's back.
- ***Rescuer B:*** Place your arms under patient's hips and calves.
- ***Rescuers A and B:***
  - Slide patient to edge of bed and bend toward him or her with your knees slightly bent.
  - Then lift and curl patient to your chests and return to standing position.
  - Rotate, and slide patient gently onto stretcher.

## ➤ 56—DIRECT GROUND LIFT

- Set stretcher in its lowest position, and place oppo-site patient.
- ***Rescuers A and B:*** Get in position along one side of patient. Rescuer A is at head-end; Rescuer B at foot-end.
- ***Rescuers A and B:*** Drop to one knee, facing patient.
- Then place patient's arms on his or her chest.
- ***Rescuer A:*** Cradle patient's head and neck by sliding one arm under the neck to grasp shoulder; place your other arm under patient's lower back.
- ***Rescuer B:*** Slide one arm under patient's knees and other under patient above buttocks.
- If a third rescuer is available, he or she should place both arms under patient's waist while Rescuers A and B slide their arms up to mid-back or down to buttocks.
- On a signal, crew lifts patient to their knees.
- On a signal, crew members stand and carry patient to stretcher, drop to one knee, and roll forward to place patient onto mattress.

➤ **57—LOADING WHEELED STRETCHER**

- Lift rear step of ambulance.
- Move stretcher as close to ambulance as possible.
- Make sure stretcher is locked in its lowest level before lifting (depends on local procedure and type of stretcher).
- ***Rescuers A and B:*** Get in position on opposite sides of stretcher, bend at knees, and grasp lower bar of stretcher frame.
- Come to a full standing position with backs straight.
- Use oblique stepping movements to move stretcher to ambulance.
- Secure stretcher into ambulance using the appropriate securing device.
- Engage both forward and rear catches to hold stretcher in place.

### ➤ 58—CRADLE CARRY

- Place one arm across patient's back with your hand under his or her arm.
- Place your other arm under his or her knees and lift.
- If patient is conscious, have him or her place nearest arm over your shoulder.

### ➤ 59—FIREFIGHTER'S DRAG

- Place patient in supine position.
- Tie patient's hands together with something that will not cut into skin.
- Straddle patient, facing his or her head.
- Crouch and pass your head through patient's trussed arms, and then raise your body to raise patient's head, neck, and upper trunk.
- Crawl on your hands and knees, dragging patient and keeping patient's head low to ground.

➤ **60—BLANKET DRAG**

- Gather half of blanket up against patient's side.
- Roll patient toward your knees.
- Gently roll patient onto blanket.
- Roll up blanket by patient's head, neck, and shoulders and drag this rolled material, keeping patient's head as low to ground as possible.

### ➤ 61—PACK STRAP CARRY

- Have patient stand.
- Turn your back to patient, bringing his or her arms over your shoulders to cross your chest.
- Keep patient's arms as straight as possible and armpits over your shoulders.
- Hold patient's wrists, bend, and pull patient onto your back.

### ➤ 62—PIGGY BACK CARRY

- Assist patient to a standing position.
- Turn your back to patient, placing patient's arms over your shoulder so the arms cross your chest.
- While patient holds on with his or her arms, crouch and grasp patient's thighs.
- Use a lifting motion to move patient onto your back.
- Pass your forearms under patient's knees and grasp his or her wrists.

## ➤ 63—FIREFIGHTER'S CARRY

- Place your toes against patient's toes, and pull patient toward you.
- Bend at waist and flex your knees.
- Duck and pull patient across your shoulder, keeping hold of one of his or her wrists.
- Use your free arm to reach between patient's legs and grasp thigh.
- Let weight of patient fall onto your shoulders.
- Stand up, transferring your grip on patient's thigh to his or her wrist.

## ➤ EFFECTS OF AGING

- *Depositing of cholesterol*—arterial walls become thicker, increasing the risk of heart attack, stroke, and hypertension.
- *Decreased cardiac output*—diminished activity and less tolerance of physical stress, making patient more prone to falls.
- *Decreased elasticity of lungs and decreased activity of cilia*—less ability to clear foreign substances from lungs, increasing risk of pneumonia.
- *Fewer taste buds, less saliva, less acid production, and slower movement in digestive system*—difficulty chewing and swallowing, less enjoyment of eating; difficulty digesting and absorbing food; increased constipation; early feeling of fullness when eating. These conditions make patient more prone to weight loss and abdominal pain.
- *Diminished liver and kidney function*—increased toxicity from alcohol and medications; diminished ability of blood to clot, which makes patient prone to bleed.
- *Decreased muscle mass and loss of minerals from bones*—decreased strength and increased risk for falls, leading to more fractures.
- *Multiple medical conditions*—high probability of many medications, sometimes prescribed by different physicians.
- *Death of friends and family*—increased risk of depression or loss of social support, which in turn increases the risk of suicide.
- *Loss of skin elasticity and shrinking of sweat glands*—thin, dry, wrinkled skin, which increases risk of injury.

## ➤ 64—DEALING WITH PEDIATRIC PATIENTS

- Take BSI precautions.
- Identify yourself (simple/informal).
- Let child know someone will call parents.
- Determine if there are life-threatening problems, and treat them immediately.
- Let child have a nearby toy.
- Kneel or sit at child's eye level.
- Make eye contact without staring.
- Smile.
- Touch child or hold his or her hand or foot if appropriate.
- Explain in simple terms equipment that you plan to use.
- Stop occasionally to confirm that child understands your actions.
- Never lie to a child.

### ➤ 65—INFANT FBAO—CONSCIOUS PATIENT

- Take BSI precautions.
- Confirm complete airway obstruction.
- Check for serious breathing difficulty, ineffective cough, and no strong cry.
- Give up to 5 back blows and 5 chest thrusts.
- Repeat back blows and chest thrusts until obstruction is expelled or infant goes unconscious.

### ➤ 66—INFANT FBAO—PATIENT BECOMES UNCONSCIOUS

- If a second rescuer is available, have him or her activate EMS.
- Open the airway, and check for breathing. If no breathing, go to the next step.
- Attempt to ventilate. If still obstructed, reposition head and chin. Then try to ventilate again.
- If ventilation is unsuccessful, administer up to 5 back blows and 5 chest thrusts.
- Open the airway with a tongue-jaw lift. If you see the object, remove it.
- Repeat the last three steps until ventilation is effective. Then continue the steps in CPR, as needed.
- If rescuer is alone and the airway obstruction is not relieved after 1 minute, activate EMS.

**\*NOTE:** *If patient is breathing or resumes effective breathing, place in recovery position.*

### ➤ 67—INFANT FBAO—UNCONSCIOUS PATIENT

- Take BSI precautions.
- Establish unresponsiveness. If second rescuer is available, have him or her activate EMS.
- Open airway, and check for breathing. If no breathing, go on to the next step.
- Attempt to ventilate. If still obstructed, reposition head and chin and try to ventilate again.
- If ventilation is unsuccessful, administer up to 5 back blows and 5 chest thrusts.
- Open the airway with a tongue-jaw lift. If you see the object, remove it.
- Repeat the last three steps until ventilation is effective. Then continue steps of CPR, as needed.
- If rescuer is alone and airway obstruction is not relieved after about 1 minute, activate EMS.

**NOTE:* *If patient is breathing or resumes effective breathing, place in recovery position.*

## ➤ 68—INFANT AND CHILD—TWO-RESCUER CPR

- Take BSI precautions.
- Establish unresponsiveness.
- Activate EMS system. Then follow these steps.

### Rescuer A:

- Open airway (heat-tilt/chin-lift or jaw-thrust). Check breathing.
- If breathing is absent/inadequate, give 2 slow breaths and ensure other signs of circulation.
- If circulation is present but breathing is absent, provide rescue breathing (1 breath every 3 seconds).

### Rescuer B:

- If no signs of circulation or heart rate is less than 60 with signs of poor perfusion, begin cycles of 5 chest compressions and 1 breath. Compression rate is 100 for children and at least 100 for infants.
- After 20 cycles of 5:1 (approximately 1 minute), provide a ventilation and then reassess for signs of a pulse and circulation.

*★NOTE: If patient is breathing or resumes breathing, place in recovery position.*

### ➤ 69—CHILD FBAO—CONSCIOUS PATIENT

- Ask: "Are you choking?" "Can you speak?"
- Give abdominal thrusts.
- Repeat thrusts until effective or patient becomes unconscious.

### ➤ 70—CHILD FBAO—PATIENT BECOMES UNCONSCIOUS

- If second rescuer is available, have him or her activate EMS system.
- Open the airway with a tongue-jaw lift. If you see object, remove it.
- Open airway and try to ventilate. If no chest rise, reopen airway and try to ventilate it again.
- If ventilation is unsuccessful, give up to 5 abdominal thrusts.
- Repeat last three steps until effective. Then provide additional steps of CPR, as needed.
- If rescuer is alone and airway obstruction is not relieved after about 1 minute, activate EMS system.

**\*NOTE:** *If patient is breathing or resumes effective breathing, replace in recovery position.*

### ➤ 71—CHILD FBAO—UNCONSCIOUS PATIENT

- Take BSI precautions.
- Establish unresponsiveness. If second rescuer is available, have him or her activate EMS system.
- Open airway, and check for breathing. If breathing is absent or inadequate, go to next step.
- Attempt to ventilate. If unsuccessful, reopen the airway and try to ventilate again.
- If ventilation is unsuccessful, give up to 5 abdominal thrusts.
- Open the airway with tongue-jaw lift. If you see object, remove it.
- Repeat last three steps until ventilation is effective. Then continue the steps of CPR, as needed.
- If rescuer is alone or airway obstruction is not relieved after about 1 minute, activate EMS system.

*✱NOTE: If patient is breathing or resumes effective breathing, place in recovery position.*

## ➤ 72—CHILD AND INFANT—ONE-RESCUER CPR

- Take BSI precautions.
- Establish unresponsiveness.
- If second rescuer is available, have him or her activate EMS.
- Open airway (head-tilt/chin-lift or jaw thrust), and check for breathing.
- If breathing is absent/inadequate, give 2 slow breaths (1 to 1.5 seconds each), and watch chest rise. If signs of circulation and pulse are present (carotid for child and brachial for infant) but no breathing, provide rescue breathing (1 breath every 3 seconds).
- If no signs of circulation or pulse rate is less than 60 with signs of poor perfusion, begin cycles of 5 compressions to 1 ventilation (compression rate of 100).
- After a minute, check for signs of circulation and pulse (carotid for child and brachial for infant). If rescuer is alone, activate EMS. If no signs of circulation or pulse is still less than 60 in the infant, continue 5:1 cycles. If signs of circulation are present but breathing is absent or inadequate, continue rescue breathing at 1 breath every 3 seconds.

*✱NOTE: If patient is breathing or resumes effective breathing, place in recovery position.*

## ➤ 73—CHILD SAFETY SEAT IMMOBILIZATION: ASSESSMENT

- Take BSI precautions.
- Then take the following steps.

### Rescuer A:

- Get in position behind patient. Apply manual in-line stabilization of head and neck. Maintain manual stabilization throughout procedure.
- Based on initial assessment and patient's status, determine if he or she should be immobilized in seat (#74) or rapidly extricated (#75).

### Rescuer B:

- Prepare equipment.
- Apply rigid extrication collar, or improvise a collar with rolled hand towel for newborn or infant.
- Place a small blanket or bath towel on child's lap. Either strap or use wide tape to secure pelvis and chest area to seat.
- Place a towel roll on both sides of head to fill voids. Tape forehead in place. Then place tape across collar or maxilla. Avoid taping chin, which would place pressure on child's neck and close airway.
- Carry patient and seat to ambulance and strap them onto stretcher with stretcher head raised.
- Reassess distal PMS.

### ➤ 74—IMMOBILIZING PATIENT IN A CHILD SAFETY SEAT

- Take BSI precautions.
- Then follow these steps.

#### *Rescuer A:*

- Stabilize child safety seat in an upright position.
- Maintain manual stabilization of head and neck throughout procedure until patient is completely immobilized.

#### *Rescuer B:*

- Prepare equipment.
- Apply rigid extrication collar, or improvise a collar with rolled hand towel for newborn or infant.
- Place a small blanket or bath towel on child's lap. Either strap or use wide tape to secure pelvis and chest area to seat.
- Place a towel roll on both sides of head to fill voids. Tape forehead in place. Then place tape across collar or maxilla. Avoid taping chin, which would place pressure on child's neck and close airway.
- Carry patient and seat to ambulance.
- Strap them onto stretcher with stretcher head raised.
- Reassess PMS.

### ➤ 75—RAPID EXTRICATION FROM CHILD SAFETY SEAT

- Take BSI precautions.
- Then follow these steps.

#### *Rescuer A:*

- Stabilize child safety seat in upright position.
- Maintain manual stabilization of head and neck throughout procedure until patient is completely immobilized.

#### *Rescuer B:*

- Prepare equipment.
- Loosen or cut car seat straps and false front guard.
- Apply rigid extrication collar, or improvise with rolled hand towel in newborn/infant.
- Place child safety seat on center of long backboard and slowly tilt it back into a supine position, being careful not to allow patient to slide out of chair. If patient has a large head, it is helpful to place a towel under area where shoulders will end up on board.

#### *Rescuer A:*

- Call for a coordinated long axis move onto board.
- Continue to maintain manual stabilization of head and neck.

#### *Rescuer B:*

- Grasp chest and axilla with each hand, and do a coordinated long axis move onto board. Make sure child is positioned at the end of board and not in the middle.

- Place a rolled blanket on each side of patient.
- Strap pelvis and upper chest to board. Do not strap abdomen down. Tape lower legs to board with wide tape.
- Place a towel roll on both sides of head to fill voids. Tape forehead in place. Then place tape across collar or maxilla. Do not tape across chin to avoid pressure on patient's neck.
- Reassess PMS.

➤ **CHARACTERISTICS OF ANATOMY AND PHYSIOLOGY**

- Tongue is larger than an adult's and more likely to block the airway.
- Smaller airway is more easily blocked.
- Abundant secretions can block the airway.
- Baby teeth are easily broken and can block the airway.
- Flat nose and face is hard to get a good mask seal.
- Big head and weak neck muscles are prone to trauma.
- Open fontanelles may indicate rising intracranial pressure (ICP) if bulging or dehydration if sunken.
- Short narrow trachea can close easily with hyperextension of the neck.
- Short neck is difficult to immobilize.
- Children tend to be abdominal breathers.
- Prolonged periods of rapid respiratory rate cause tiring and ultimately lead to respiratory distress.
- Larger body surface area (BSA) makes the patient prone to hypothermia.
- Thinner skin is more sensitive to burns.
- Softer bones are more flexible, which when injured result in fewer fractures and more internal damage.
- Spleen and liver are more exposed, which makes them more prone to injury.
- Infants are primarily nose breathers.

### ➤ DEVELOPMENTAL CHARACTERISTICS

#### *Newborns and Infants—Birth to 1 Year*

- Do not like to be separated from parents.
- Minimal stranger anxiety.
- Used to being undressed, but like to feel warm.
- Follow movements with eyes.
- Do not want to be "suffocated" by oxygen mask.

#### *Toddlers—1 to 3 Years*

- Do not like to be touched or separated from parents.
- Believe their illness is a punishment for being bad.
- Do not like having clothing removed.
- Frighten easily and overreact.
- Have begun to assert independence.
- Do not want to be "suffocated" by oxygen mask.

#### *Preschool—3 to 5 Years*

- Do not like to be touched or separated from parents.
- Modest and do not like clothing removed.
- Believe that their illness is a punishment for being bad.
- Fear of blood, pain, and permanent injury.
- Curious, communicative, and can be cooperative.
- Do not want to be "suffocated" by an oxygen mask.

#### *School Age—6 to 10 Years*

- Cooperative but like opinions heard.
- Fear blood, pain, disfigurement, and permanent injury.
- Modest and do not like their bodies exposed.

*(continued)*

### *Adolescents—11 to 18 Years*

- Want to be treated as adults.
- Feel they are indestructible, but may have fears of permanent injury and disfigurement.
- Vary in emotional and physical development and may not be comfortable with their changing bodies.

### ➤ ADDITIONAL SIGNIFICANT MOI FOR A CHILD

- Falls from more than 10 feet.
- Bicycle collision.
- Vehicle in medium-speed collision.

> ### STAGES OF LABOR

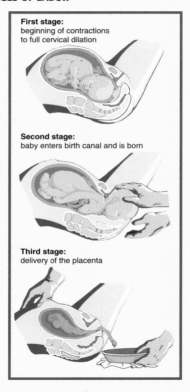

**First stage:**
beginning of contractions
to full cervical dilation

**Second stage:**
baby enters birth canal and is born

**Third stage:**
delivery of the placenta

### ➤ 76—ASSESSMENT OF MOTHER FOR IMMINENT DELIVERY

- Take BSI precautions.
- Conduct an initial assessment.
- Obtain mother's history to determine active labor. History includes:
  - Length of term.
  - Number of previous pregnancies and births.
  - Frequency and duration of uterine contractions.
  - Recent vaginal discharge or hemorrhage.
  - Whether or not "water broke" yet.
  - Presence of strain or urge to move bowels.
- With mother's permission, examine for crowning.
- Feel for uterine contractions when mother says she is having one.
- Take a set of vitals and make decision: prepare for delivery or begin transport.

➤ **NEWBORN RESUSCITATION**

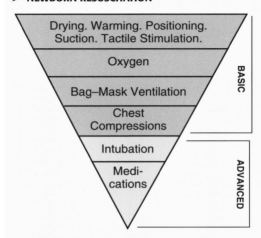

| APGAR SCORE | | Points | Score | |
|---|---|---|---|---|
| | | | 1 min | 5 min |
| **A** | APPEARANCE (SKIN COLOR) | | | |
| | Blue or pale extremities | 0 | | |
| | Pink trunk and blue extremities | 1 | | |
| | Completely pink | 2 | _____ | _____ |
| **P** | PULSE | | | |
| | Absent | 0 | | |
| | < 100 | 1 | | |
| | > 100 | 2 | _____ | _____ |
| **G** | GRIMACE (IRRITABILITY) | | | |
| | No response | 0 | | |
| | Grimace or whimpers | 1 | | |
| | Actively cries | 2 | _____ | _____ |
| **A** | ACTIVITY (MUSCLE TONE) | | | |
| | Flaccid, limp | 0 | | |
| | Some flexion of extremities | 1 | | |
| | Active extremity motion | 2 | _____ | _____ |
| **R** | RESPIRATORY EFFORT | | | |
| | Absent | 0 | | |
| | Slow and irregular | 1 | | |
| | Strong cry | 2 | _____ | _____ |

**TOTAL SCORE**  _____

*(continued)*

Ideally scores are taken at one and five minutes after birth. If the neonate is not breathing, DO NOT withhold resuscitation for an APGAR score. Total scores indicate the following:

7–10   indicates an active and vigorous neonate who requires routine care.

4–6   indicates a moderately depressed neonate who requires oxygenation and stimulation.

0–3   indicates a severely depressed neonate who requires immediate resuscitation.

By assessing the APGAR score at one minute and repeating at five minutes, it is possible to determine whether or not intervention has caused a change in the neonate's status.

### ➤ 77—MANAGEMENT OF ABSORBED POISONS

- Size up situation, and take the necessary precautions to prevent injury to yourself and your crew.
- Remove patient from source. Avoid contaminating yourself with poison.
- Conduct an initial assessment.
- Maintain an open airway.
- Administer high-concentration oxygen.
- Perform a focused history and physical exam, including SAMPLE history and vital signs.
- Brush powders from patient. Be careful not to abrade patient's skin.
- Remove contaminated clothing and other articles, such as shoes and jewelry.
- Quickly gather information about product.
- If appropriate, irrigate with large amounts of clear water for at least 20 minutes. Call medical direction.
- Perform ongoing assessment.
- Be alert for shock, and transport as soon as possible.

### ➤ 78—MANAGEMENT OF INGESTED POISONS (EMT-B SKILL)

- Take BSI precautions.
- Conduct an initial assessment.
- Maintain an open airway.
- Perform a focused history and physical exam, including SAMPLE history and vital signs.
- Quickly gather information about substance.
- Call medical direction on scene or en route.
- If directed, administer activated charcoal.
- Position patient for vomiting and save all vomitus. Have suction ready.
- Perform ongoing assessment.
- Transport as soon as possible.

## ➤ 79—MANAGEMENT OF INHALED POISONS

- Size-up the situation, and take the necessary precautions to prevent injury to yourself and your crew.*
- Remove patient from the source. Avoid contaminating yourself with poison.
- Maintain open airway. Stay alert for vomiting. Properly position the patient and have suction equipment ready.
- Conduct an initial assessment.
- Administer high-concentration oxygen by nonrebreather mask.
- Perform a focused history and physical exam, including a SAMPLE history.
- Remove contaminated clothing and other articles (e.g., shoes, jewelry).
- Assess baseline vital signs.
- Quickly gather information about product (containers, bottles, and labels).
- Call medical direction on scene or en route.
- Transport as soon as possible.
- Perform ongoing assessment en route.

*SAFETY NOTE: In the presence of hazardous fumes or gases, wear protective clothing and a self-contained breathing apparatus or wait for those who are properly trained and equipped to enter scene and remove patient to a safe area.*

➤ **CLASSIFICATION OF BURNS BY DEPTH**

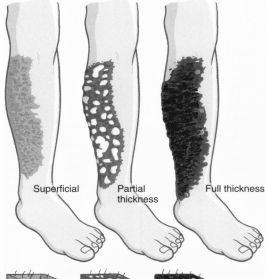

Superficial

Partial thickness

Full thickness

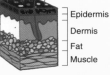

Epidermis
Dermis
Fat
Muscle

Skin reddened

Blisters

Charring

> ## RULE OF NINES—ADULTS

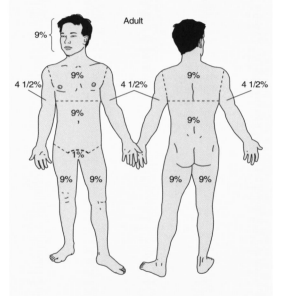

## ➤ RULE OF NINES—INFANTS AND CHILDREN

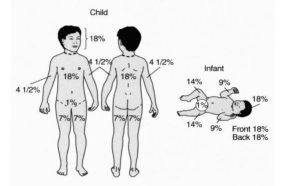

Child

18%

4 1/2%    18%    4 1/2%

4 1/2%

1%

7% 7%

18%

4 1/2%

7% 7%

Infant

14%    9%

1%

14%    9%    18%

Front 18%
Back 18%

### ➤ CLASSIFICATION OF BURN SEVERITY

#### *Minor Burns—Adults*
- Full-thickness burns <2 percent, excluding face, hands, feet, genitalia, or respiratory tract.
- Partial-thickness burns <15 percent.
- Superficial burns of 50 percent or less.

#### *Minor Burns—Children <5 yrs. old*
- Partial-thickness burns of <10 percent of body surface.

#### *Moderate Burns—Adults*
- Full-thickness burns of 2–10 percent, excluding face, hands, feet, genitalia, or respiratory tract.
- Partial-thickness burns of 15–30 percent.
- Superficial burns that involve more than 50 percent body surface.

#### *Moderate Burns—Children <5 yrs. old*
- Partial-thickness burns of 10–20 percent of body surface.

#### *Critical Burns—Adults*
- All burns complicated by injuries of respiratory tract, other soft-tissue injuries, and bone injuries.
- Partial- or full-thickness burns of face, feet, hands, genitalia, or respiratory tract.
- Full-thickness burns of >10 percent.
- Partial-thickness burns of >30 percent.
- Burns complicated by musculoskeletal injuries.
- Circumferential burns.

*(continued)*

### *Critical Burns—Children <5 yrs. old*

- Full-thickness or partial-thickness burns of >20 percent of body surface.

## ➤ 80—ACTIVE RAPID REWARMING OF FROZEN PARTS

- Take BSI precautions.
- Conduct an initial assessment.
- Conduct focused history and physical exam, including taking baseline vital signs.
- Consider administering oxygen by nonrebreather mask.
- Heat water to a temperature between 100°F and 105°F.
- Fill container with heated water and prepare injured part by removing clothing, jewelry, bands, or straps.
- Fully immerse injured part. Do not allow injured area to touch sides or bottom of container. Do not place any pressure on affected part. Continuously stir the water. When water cools below 100°F, remove affected part and add more warm water. The patient may complain of moderate pain as the affected area rewarms or may experience periods of intense pain.
- If you complete rewarming of the part, gently dry the affected area and apply a dry sterile dressing.
- Place dry sterile dressings between fingers and toes before dressing hands/feet.
- Cover the site with blankets or whatever is available to keep affected area warm. Do not allow these coverings to come in contact with injured area or to put pressure on site.
- Keep patient at rest. Do not allow patient to walk if a lower extremity has been frostbitten or frozen.
- Keep entire patient warm.
- Continue to monitor the patient.

*(continued)*

- Assist circulation according to local protocol. (Some systems recommend rhythmically and carefully raising and lowering affected limb.)
- Do not allow limb to refreeze.
- Transport patient as soon as possible, with affected limb slightly elevated.

## ➤ 81—PATIENT REFUSAL PROCEDURE

- Spend time effectively communicating with patient (includes reasoning, persistence, and strategies to convince patient to go to hospital).
- Clearly inform patient of consequences of not going to hospital.
- Consult with medical direction.
- Contact family to help convince patient.
- Call law enforcement who may be able to order or "arrest" serious patient in order to force patient to go to hospital.
- Try to determine why patient is refusing care.
- Complete thorough documentation of refusal, have patient sign refusal release, and have witness sign the release (e.g., bystander, police, family).

*NOTE: Procedure may differ by state and jurisdiction. Always follow your medical director's advice.*

### ➤ 82—HANDWASHING

- Remove watch and rings. Roll up sleeves.
- Adjust water flow and temperature.
- Wet hands and distal forearms.
- Dispense soap onto hands.
- Scrub lower arms and hands. Clean around and under nails.
- Rinse thoroughly under running water to remove all soap. Do not touch sink!
- Use a paper towel to shut off faucet in order to avoid re-contaminating hands.

**NOTE:** *Even though you wear protective gloves with your patients, handwashing must still be performed immediately after each call.*

### ➤ 83—TRANSFERRING THE PATIENT

- Take BSI precautions.
- Transfer patient as soon as possible. In a routine admission or when an illness or injury is not life-threatening, first check to see what is to be done with patient.
- A rescuer should remain with patient until transfer is complete.
- Assist emergency department staff as required.
- Give a complete verbal report of patient's condition and treatment administered.
- Complete your prehospital care report and turn a copy over to hospital staff.
- Transfer patient's personal effects.
- Obtain your release from hospital, if required in your region.

### ➤ 84—ACTIONS TO BE TAKEN AT HOSPITAL

- Take BSI precautions.
- Clean ambulance interior as required by your service exposure control plan.
- Replace respiratory equipment as required.
- Replace disposable items according to local policies.
- Exchange equipment according to local policies.
- Make up ambulance stretcher.

### ➤ 85—TERMINATION OF ACTIVITIES IN QUARTERS

- Place contaminated linens in biohazard container and non-contaminated linens in regular hamper.
- Remove and clean patient care equipment as required.
- Clean and sanitize respiratory equipment as needed.
- Clean and sanitize ambulance interior as required. Use germicide on devices and surfaces that were in contact with blood and body fluids.
- Wash thoroughly and change soiled clothing.
- Replace expendable supplies and equipment as required.

### ➤ 86—CLEANING AND DISINFECTING EQUIPMENT

- Use *low-level disinfectant*—one approved by the EPA, such as Lysol®, to clean and kill germs on ambulance floors and walls.
- Use *intermediate-level disinfectant*—such as a mixture of 1:100 bleach-to-water to clean and kill germs on equipment.
- Use *high-level disinfectant*—such as Cidex Plus®, to destroy all forms of microbial life except high numbers of bacterial spores.

**✱*NOTE: Sterilization is required to destroy all possible sources of infection on equipment that will be used invasively.*

## ➤ DANGEROUS AREAS NEAR A HELICOPTER

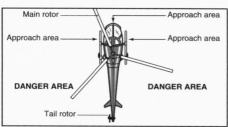

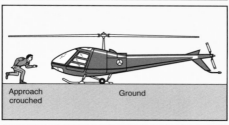

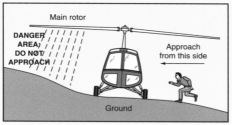

### ➤ 87—ESTABLISHING COMMAND AT A MULTIPLE-CASUALTY INCIDENT (MCI)

- Perform a scene size-up.
- Locate police and fire officers and establish a unified command post.
- Don EMS command vest.
- Notify EMS dispatcher:
  - Declare an MCI.
  - Indicate extent of incident.
  - Note whether ongoing or contained.
  - Estimate number of patients.
  - Identify location of command post.
  - Request number of BLS/ALS units.
- Designate a triage officer.
- Designate a staging officer:
  - Select location for staging sector.
  - Notify dispatcher to have all additional ambulances respond to staging.
- Request dispatcher roll call hospitals for bed availability.
- Designate treatment officer and location for this sector (as needed).
- Designate transportation officer and location for this sector (as needed).
  - Consider need for aeromedical evacuation and appropriate landing zone nearby scene.
  - Consider usefulness of a school bus to transport walking wounded (low-priority) patients. Make sure everyone on bus is medically examined and that medical personnel also ride bus.

*(continued)*

133

- Consider need for extrication sector (if not already established).
- Consider need for a safety officer (as needed).
- Consider need for a follow-up CISD and rehab of personnel.
- Keep dispatcher and other service chiefs in close contact throughout incident.
- Along with police and fire officers, consider need for a public information officer to work with arriving media.

## ➤ MCI TERMS AND DEFINITIONS

*EMS operations*—the person who is responsible for the actual operations of the incident.

*IMS*—incident management system.

*MCI*—multiple-casualty incident.

*Rehab sector*—the location where emergency service providers are sent to be rehydrated, cooled off, and to obtain rest and medical monitoring of vital signs if needed.

*Safety officer*—the person assigned at large-scale incidents to ensure safety of all EMS personnel at the scene.

*Singular command*—single agency controls all resources and operations at an MCI.

*Staging sector*—the dedicated area where resources including personnel, vehicles, and equipment are held until needed on scene.

*Transport sector*—an area established for ambulance loading and supervised patient evacuation. The destinations of all patients are logged here.

*Treatment sector*—a designated area set up to treat patients prior to transport.

*Triage sector*—an area established for reassessment and removal of patients for a treatment sector.

*Triage*—sorting or setting priorities for patient treatment.

*Unified command*—the commanding officers from each public safety agency working together to make key decisions at an MCI.

> **PATIENT TRIAGE PRIORITIES**

*P–1:* Treatable life-threatening illness or injuries, including airway and breathing difficulties, uncontrolled or severe bleeding, decreased mental status, patients with severe medical problems, shock, severe burns. (Red-colored designation)

*P–2:* Serious but not life-threatening illness or injuries including burns without airway problems, major or multiple bone or joint injuries, back injuries with or without spinal-cord damage. (Yellow-colored designation)

*P–3:* "Walking wounded" including minor musculoskeletal injuries, minor soft-tissue injuries. (Green-colored designation)

*P–4: (sometimes called Priority—0):* Dead or fatally injured, including exposed brain matter, cardiac arrest (no pulse for over 20 minutes, except with cold-water drowning or severe hypothermia), decapitation, severed trunk, and incineration. (Black-colored designation)

# ➤ MUSCULOSKELETAL SYSTEM

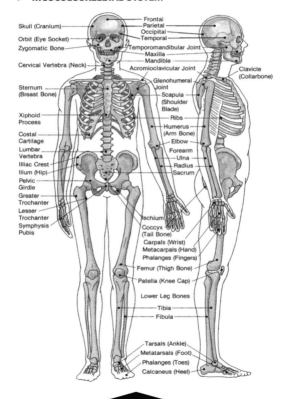

Skull (Cranium)
Orbit (Eye Socket)
Zygomatic Bone
Cervical Vertebra (Neck)
Sternum (Breast Bone)
Xiphoid Process
Costal Cartilage
Lumbar Vertebra
Iliac Crest
Ilium (Hip)
Pelvic Girdle
Greater Trochanter
Lesser Trochanter
Symphysis Pubis

Frontal
Parietal
Occipital
Temporal
Temporomandibular Joint
Maxilla
Mandible
Acromioclavicular Joint
Glenohumeral Joint
Scapula (Shoulder Blade)
Ribs
Humerus (Arm Bone)
Elbow
Forearm
Ulna
Radius
Sacrum

Clavicle (Collarbone)

Ischium
Coccyx (Tail Bone)
Carpals (Wrist)
Metacarpals (Hand)
Phalanges (Fingers)
Femur (Thigh Bone)
Patella (Knee Cap)

Lower Leg Bones
Tibia
Fibula

Tarsals (Ankle)
Metatarsals (Foot)
Phalanges (Toes)
Calcaneus (Heel)

## ➤ NERVOUS SYSTEM

**The Brain**

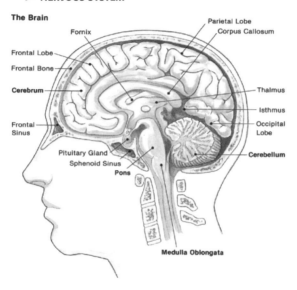

Fornix

Parietal Lobe
Corpus Callosum

Frontal Lobe

Frontal Bone

Cerebrum

Thalmus

Isthmus

Frontal
Sinus

Occipital
Lobe

Pituitary Gland

Cerebellum

Sphenoid Sinus

**Pons**

Medulla Oblongata

## ➤ DIVISIONS OF THE SPINAL CORD

**Divisions of the
Spinal Cord**

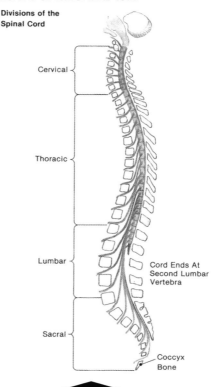

Cervical

Thoracic

Lumbar

Cord Ends At
Second Lumbar
Vertebra

Sacral

Coccyx
Bone

➤ **CRANIAL HEMATOMAS**

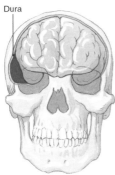

Dura

Subdural

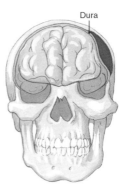

Dura

Epidural

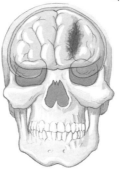

Intracerebral

## ➤ DIGESTIVE SYSTEM

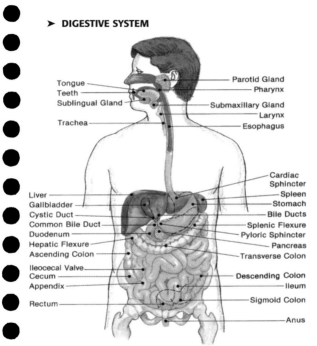

### ➤ URINARY SYSTEM

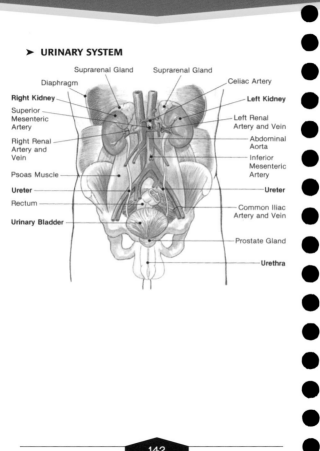

### ➤ RELATED TERMS

*Indications*—specific signs, symptoms, or circumstances under which it is appropriate to administer a drug to a patient.

*Contraindications*—specific signs, symptoms, or circumstances under which it is not appropriate, and may be harmful, to administer a drug to the patient.

*Side effect*—any action of a drug other than the desired action.

### ➤ DRUG ADMINISTRATION PROCEDURE

Before administering a drug:
1. Confirm the order.
2. Write it down.
3. Check "five rights":
   • Do I have the right patient?
   • Is this the right medication?
   • Is this the right dose?
   • Is this the right time for the medication to be given?
   • Am I giving this medication by the right route of administration?

### ➤ ACTIVATED CHARCOAL

#### Medication Name

- Generic: activated charcoal.
- Trade: SuperChar, InstaChar, Actidose, Liqui-Char, and others.

#### Indications

- Poisoning by mouth.

#### Contraindications

- Altered mental status.
- Ingestion of acids or alkalis.
- Inability to swallow.

#### Medication Form

- Pre-mixed in water, frequently available in plastic bottle containing 12.5 grams of activated charcoal.
- Powder—should be avoided in field.

#### Dosage

- Adults and children: 1 gram activated charcoal/kg of body weight.
- Usual adult dose: 25–50 grams.
- Usual pediatric dose: 12.5–25 grams.

#### Administration

- Consult medical direction.
- Shake container thoroughly.
- Since medication looks like mud, patient may need to be persuaded to drink it. Providing a covered container and a straw will prevent patient from seeing the medication and so may improve patient compliance.

*(continued)*

- If patient does not drink the medication right away, the charcoal will settle. Shake or stir it again before administering.
- Record the name, dose, route, and time of administration of the medication.

### Actions

- Activated charcoal absorbs (binds) certain poisons and prevents them from being absorbed into the body.
- Not all brands of activated charcoal are the same: some absorb much more than others, so consult medical direction about the brand to use.

### Side Effects

- Black stools.
- Some patients, particularly those who have ingested poisons that cause nausea, may vomit. If patient vomits, repeat the dose once.

### Reassessment Strategies

- Be prepared for the patient to vomit or to deteriorate further.

### ➤ EPINEPHRINE AUTO-INJECTOR

#### *Medication Name*

- Generic: epinephrine.
- Trade: Adrenalin.
- Delivery system: EpiPen® or EpiPen® Jr.

#### *Indications*

Must meet the following three criteria:

- Patient exhibits signs of a severe allergic reaction, including either respiratory distress or shock.
- Medication is prescribed for this patient by a physician.
- Medical direction authorizes use for this patient.

#### *Contraindications*

- No contraindications when used in a life-threatening situation.

#### *Medication Form*

- Liquid administered by an auto-injector (an automatically injectable needle-and-syringe system).

#### *Dosage*

- Adults: one adult auto-injector (0.3 mg).
- Infant and child: one infant/child auto-injector (0.15 mg).

*(continued)*

### Administration

- Obtain patient's prescribed auto-injector. Ensure prescription is written for the patient who is experiencing the severe allergic reaction. Ensure medication is not discolored (if visible).
- Obtain order from medical direction, either on-line or off-line.
- Remove cap from auto-injector. Place tip of auto-injector against patient's thigh (lateral portion, midway between waist and knee).
- Push the injector firmly against the thigh until the injector activates.
- Hold the injector in place until the medication is injected (at least 10 seconds).
- Record activity and time.
- Dispose of injector in biohazard container.

### Actions

- Dilates the bronchioles.
- Constricts blood vessels.

### Side Effects

- Increased heart rate.
- Pallor.
- Dizziness.
- Chest pain.
- Headache.
- Nausea, vomiting.
- Excitability, anxiety.

*(continued)*

147

### Reassessment Strategies

- Transport.
- Continue focused assessment of airway, breathing, and circulatory status.
- If patient's condition continues to worsen (decreasing mental status, increased breathing difficulty, decreasing blood pressure):
  - Obtain medical direction for an additional dose of epinephrine.
  - Treat for shock.
  - Prepare to initiate basic life support procedures (CPR, AED).
- If patient's condition improves, provide supportive care. That is, continue oxygen and treat for shock.

## ➤ NITROGLYCERIN

### *Medication Name*

- Generic: nitroglycerin.
- Trade: Nitrostat, Nitrolingual Spray.

### *Indications*

All of the following conditions must be met:
- Patient complains of chest pain.
- Patient with history of cardiac problems.
- Patient's physician has prescribed nitroglycerin (NTG).
- Systolic blood pressure is greater than 100.
- Medical direction authorizes administration of the medication.

### *Contraindications*

- Patient has hypotension or a systolic blood pressure below 100.
- Patient has a head injury.
- Patient is an infant or child.
- Patient has already taken the maximum prescribed dose.

### *Medication Form*

- Tablet, sublingual spray.

### *Dosage*

- One dose, repeat in five minutes. If no relief, if systolic blood pressure remains above 100, and if authorized by medical direction, up to a maximum of three doses.

*(continued)*

### Administration

- Perform focused assessment for cardiac patient.
- Take blood pressure. (Systolic pressure must be above 100.)
- Contact medical direction if no standing orders.
- Assure right medication, right patient, right dose, right route, right time.
- Check expiration date.
- Assure patient is alert.
- Question patient on last dose taken and effects.
- Assure understanding of route of administration.
- Ask patient to lift tongue. Place tablet or spray dose under it (while wearing gloves), or have patient place tablet or spray under it.
- Have patient keep mouth closed with tablet under tongue (without swallowing) until dissolved and absorbed.
- Recheck blood pressure within two minutes.
- Record administration, route, and time.
- Perform reassessment.

### Actions

- Relaxes blood vessels.
- Decreases workload of heart.

### Side Effects

- Hypotension (lowers blood pressure).
- Headache.
- Pulse rate changes.

*(continued)*

### *Reassessment Strategies*

- Monitor blood pressure.
- Ask patient about effect on pain relief.
- Seek medical direction before readministration.
- Record assessments.

### ➤ ORAL GLUCOSE

#### Medication Name

- Generic: Glucose, oral.
- Trade: Glutose, Insta-glucose.

#### Indications

- Altered mental status with a known history of diabetes mellitus.

#### Contraindications

- Unresponsiveness.
- Known diabetic has not taken insulin for days.
- Inability to swallow.

#### Medication Form

- Gel, in toothpaste-type tubes.

#### Dosage

- One tube.

#### Administration

- Assure signs and symptoms of altered mental status with a known history of diabetes.
- Assure patient is awake with a gag reflex.
- Administer glucose:
  - Place on tongue depressor between cheek and gum.
  - Self-administered between cheek and gum.
  - Perform ongoing assessment.

*(continued)*

### *Actions*

- Increases blood sugar.

### *Side Effects*

- None when given properly. May be aspirated by the patient without a gag reflex.

### *Reassessment Strategies*

- If patient loses consciousness or seizes, remove tongue depressor from mouth.

> ### PRESCRIBED INHALER

#### *Medication Name*

- Generic: albuterol, isoetharine, metaproterenol.
- Trade: Proventil, Ventolin, Bronkosol, Bronkometer, Alupent, Metaprel.

#### *Indications*

Meets all of the following criteria:
- Patient exhibits signs and symptoms of respiratory emergency.
- Patient has physician-prescribed, hand-held inhaler.
- Medical direction gives specific authorization to use.

#### *Contraindications*

- Patient is unable to use device (e.g., not alert).
- Inhaler is not prescribed for patient.
- No permission has been given by medical direction.
- Patient has already taken maximum prescribed dose prior to EMT-B's arrival.

#### *Medication Form*

- Hand-held metered dose inhaler.

#### *Dosage*

- Number of inhalations based on medical director's order or physician's order.

#### *Administration*

- Obtain order from medical direction, either on-line or off-line.
- Assure right patient, right medication, right dose, right route, right time, and patient alert enough to use inhaler. *(continued)*

- Check expiration date of inhaler.
- Check if patient has already taken any doses.
- Assure inhaler is at room temperature or warmer.
- Shake inhaler vigorously several times.
- Have patient exhale deeply.
- Have patient put lips around opening of inhaler.
- Have patient depress the hand-held inhaler as he or she begins to inhale deeply.
- Instruct patient to hold breath for as long as comfortable so medication can be absorbed.
- Put oxygen back on patient.
- Allow patient to breathe a few times, and repeat second dose if so ordered by medical direction.
- If patient has a spacer device for inhaler, it should be used.

### Actions

- Beta agonist bronchodilator dilates bronchioles, reducing airway resistance.

### Side Effects

- Increased pulse rate.
- Tremors.
- Nervousness.

### Reassessment Strategies

- Gather vital signs.
- Perform focused reassessment of chest and respiratory function.
- Observe for deterioration of patient; if breathing becomes inadequate, provide artificial respirations.

The medications listed in this section are commonly used by patients. Generic names are in lower case; trade names are capitalized and in bold-face type.

The class of each medication is listed. These classes are described below; a list of "meds" follows.

> ## CLASSES OF MEDICATIONS

**Ace Inhibitor**—relaxes arteries and promotes renal excretion of salt and water.

**Acid/Peptic**—controls excessive acid in the stomach.

**Analgesic**—relieves pain.

**Anorexiant**—reduces appetite.

**Antianginal**—prevents or relieves angina pectoris.

**Antianxiety**—prevents or reduces anxiety.

**Antiarrhythmic**—counteracts or prevents cardiac dysrhythmias.

**Antiasthmatic**—relieves the symptoms of asthma.

**Antibiotic**—helps destroy microorganisms or inhibit their growth.

**Anticoagulant**—prevents clotting of the blood.

**Antidepressant**—helps to control depression.

**Antidiabetic**—regulates blood sugar levels.

**Antifungal**—destroys or controls fungus.

**Antigout**—controls symptoms of gout.

**Antihypertensive**—controls high BP.

**Antimicrobial**—kills or inhibits the growth of microorganisms.

**Antimigraine**—prevents or controls migraine headaches.

**Antineoplastic**—prevents the spread of neoplasms or malignant cells.

**Antiprotozoal**—kills protozoa.

**Antipruritic**—relieves itching.

**Antitussive**—helps to suppress coughing.

**Antiviral**—helps to prevent or control the spread of viruses.

**Beta Blocker**—prevents beta receptor site stimulation.

**Blood Glucose Regulator**—controls blood sugar levels.

**Bronchodilator**—opens up the constricted bronchial tree.

**Calcium Channel Blocker**—inhibits the transfer of calcium in smooth muscle cells.

**Cephalosporin**—a type of antibiotic.

**CNS Stimulant**—stimulates activity of brain and spinal cord.

**Contraceptive**—prevents conception or sperm and egg uniting.

**Coronary Vasodilator**—dilates the coronary vessels.

**Corticosteriod**—adrenal cortex steroid used as for anti-inflammatory purposes.

**Decongestant**—relieves congestion of mucous membranes.

**Diuretic**—helps the body off-load water by stimulating kidneys.

**Electrolytes**—solutions that contain electrically charged ions used by the body.

**Expectorant**—promotes discharge of mucous from the respiratory tract.

**Hormones**—replace or alter endocrine system function.

**NSAID (non-steroidal anti-inflammatory drug)**—controls muscular inflammation and pain.

**Penicillin**—commonly used antibiotic substance.

**Progestin**—female sex steroid hormone.

**Sedative Hypnotic**—relaxes, calms, or tranquilizes a patient.

**Skeletal Muscle Relaxant**—calms muscle shaking, twitching, and spasm.

**Sulfonamide**—a type of antibiotic.

**Tetracycline**—a type of antibiotic.

**Vitamins**—substances found in foods that are necessary for body functions.

### ➤ THE "MEDS"

**acetaminophen**—analgesic, antipyretic
**acetaminophen codeine phosphate**—analgesic
**acetaminophen hydrocodone bitartrate**—analgesic
**acetaminophen oxycodone hydrochloride**—analgesic
**acetaminophen propoxyphene napsylate**—analgesic
**acyclovir**—antiviral
**Adalat**—antihypertensive
**Adapin**—antidepressant, antianxiety
**albuterol**—bronchodilator, antiasthmatic
**Aldomet**—antihypertensive
**allopurinol**—antigout
**alprazolam**—antianxiety, sedative hypnotic
**aminophylline**—bronchodilator
**amitriptyline**—antidepressant
**amoxapine**—antidepressant
**amoxicillin**—penicillin, antibiotic
**Amoxil**—penicillin, antibiotic
**Anacin-3**—analgesic
**Anafranil**—antidepressant
**Anaprox**—analgesic, NSAID, antiarthritic
**Anaprox DS**—analgesic, antiarthritic, NSAID
**Antivert**—antihistimine, vertigo, motion sickness
**Apresoline**—antihypertensive
**Aristocort**—corticosteriod, antiasthmatic, sulfonamide
**Asendin**—antidepressant
**aspirin**—analgesic
**Astramorph/PF**—analgesic

**Atarax**—antihistimine, antipruritic, sedative
**atenolol**—antianginal, antihypertensive, beta blocker
**Ativan**—antianxiety, sedative hypnotic
**Aventyl**—antidepressant
**Azmacort**—inhaled corticosteriod, antiasthmatic

**Bactrim**—sulfonamide, antimicrobial
**Barbita**—anticonvulsant
**benzonatate**—antitussant
**Brethaire**—bronchodilator
**Brethine**—bronchodilator
**Bricanyl**—bronchodilator
**Bronkometer**—bronchodilator
**Bronkosol**—bronchodilator
**bupropion**—antidepressant

**Calan**—antiarrhythmic, antihypertensive
**Calan SR**—antiarrhythmic, antihypertensive
**Capoten**—antihypertensive, ace inhibitor
**captopril**—antihypertensive, ace inhibitor
**carisoprodol**—skeletal muscle relaxant
**carbamazepine**—anticonvulsant
**Catapres**—antihypertensive
**cephalexin**—antibiotic, antimicrobial
**chlorpropamide**—antidiabetic
**cimetidine**—acid/peptic disorder
**clomipramine**—antidepressant
**clonazepama**—anticonvulsant
**clonidine**—antihypertensive
**codeine**—analgesic

**codeine phosphate promethazine hydrochloride**—antitussive, expectorant

**Coumadin**—anticoagulant

**Cycrin**—antineoplastic, progestin, contraceptive

**cyclobenzaprine hydrochloride**—skeletal muscle relaxant

**Darvocet-N**—analgesic

**Darvon**—analgesic

**Deltasone**—corticosteroids, antiarthritic, antineoplastic

**Depakene**—anticonvulsant

**desipramine**—antidepressant

**Desyrel**—antianxiety, antidepressant

**DiaBeta**—antidiabetic, blood glucose regulator

**Diabinese**—antidiabetic

**diazepam**—antianxiety, anticonvulsant, skeletal muscle relaxant

**diclofenac**—analgesic, antiarthritic, NSAID

**digoxin**—antiarrhythmic, cardiac glycoside

**Dilantin**—anticonvulsant

**doxepin**—antidepressant

**doxepin hydrochloride**—antianxiety, antidepressant

**doxycycline**—antibiotic, antimicrobial

**Duramorph**—analgesic

**Dyazide**—antihypertensive, diuretic

**Dynacin**—tetracycline

**Ecotrin**—analgesic

**Elavil**—antidepressant

**Elixophyllin**—antiasthmatic

**Emprin**—analgesic
**Epitol**—anticonvulsant
**Esidrix**—antihypertensive
**estrogen**—hormone
**Excedrin IS**—analgesic

**Fastin**—anorexiant
**Flagyl**—antibacterial, antiprotozoal
**Flexeril**—skeletal muscle relaxant
**fluoxetine**—antidepressant
**folic acid**—vitamin
**Folvite**—anemia, vitamin
**furosemide**—antihypertensive, diuretic

**gemfibrozil**—antilipemic
**glipizide**—antidiabetic
**Glucophage**—antidiabetic
**Glucotrol**—blood glucose regulator
**Glucotrol XL**—blood glucose regulator
**glyburide**—antidiabetic, blood glucose regulator
**Glynase Prestab**—antidiabetic, blood glucose regulator
**guaifenesin phenylpropanolamine hychloride**—antitussive, expectorant, decongestant
**guanabenz**—antihypertensive

**Humulin**—antidiabetic
**hydralazine**—antihypertensive
**hydrochlorothiazide**—antihypertensive
**hydrochlorothiazide triamterene**—antihypertensive, diuretic

**Hydrodiuril**—antihypertensive
**hydroxyzine hydrochloride**—antianxiety, antihistimine, antipruritics, sedative hypnotic

**ibuprofen**—NSAID, antiarthritic, analgesic, antipyretic
**Imdur**—antianginal, coronary vasodilator
**imipramine hydrochloride**—antidepressant
**indapamide**—antihypertensive, diuretic
**Inderal**—antianginal, antiarrhythmic, antihypertensive, antimigraine, beta blocker
**Indocin**—antiarthritic, antigout
**indomethacin**—antiarthritic, NSAID, antigout
**insulin**—antidiabetic
**Ionamin**—anorexiant
**Ismo**—antianginal, coronary vasodilator
**isoetharine**—bronchodilator
**Isoptin**—antiarrhythmic, antiarthritic, antianginal, antihypertensive, calcium channel blocker
**Isoptin SR**—antiarrhythmic, antiarthritic, antianginal, antihypertensive, calcium channel blocker
**isosorbide mononitrate**—antianginal, coronary vasodilator

**Janimine**—antidepressant

**K-Dur**—electrolyte, water balance, mineral
**Keflex**—cephalosporin
**Kenalog**—corticosteroid
**Klonopin**—anticonvulsant
**K-Tab**—electrolyte, water balance, mineral

**Lanoxin**—antiarrhythmic, cardiac glycoside
**Lanoxicaps**—antiarrhythmic, cardiac glycoside
**Larotid**—penicillin
**Lasix**—antihypertensive, diuretic
**Lopid**—antilipemic
**Lopressor**—antianginal, antihypertensive, beta blocker
**Lopurin**—antigout
**lorazepam**—antianxiety, sedative hypnotic
**Lorcet**—analgesic
**Lozol**—antihypertensive, diuretic
**Luminal**—antianxiety, anticonvulsant, sedative hypnotic, anticonvulsant

**Maxzide**—antihypertensive, diuretic
**Mazepine**—anticonvulsant
**meclizine hydrochloride**—antihistimine, vertigo, motion sickness
**medroxyprogesterone acetate**—contraceptive, progestin
**metformin**—antidiabetic
**methyldopa**—antihypertensive
**methylphenidate hydrochloride**—CNS stimulant
**Meticorten**—corticosteroids, antiarthritic
**Metoclopramide hydrochloride**—antiemetic, acid/peptic, motion sickness
**metoprolol tartrate**—antianginal, antihypertensive, beta blocker
**metronidazole**—antibacterial, antiprotozoal
**Micro-K**—electrolye, water balance
**Micronase**—antidiabetic, blood glucose regulator

**Minocin**—tetracycline
**minocycline hydrochloride**—tetracycline
**Monoket**—antianginal, coronary vasodilator
**Motrin**—analgesic, NSAID, antiarthritic, antipyretic
**MS Contin**—analgesic
**Mysoline**—anticonvulsant

**nalbuphine**—analgesic
**Naprosyn**—analgesic, antiarthritic, NSAID
**naproxen**—analgesic, antiarthritic, NSAID
**Nasacort**—corticosteriod, antiasthmatic
**nefazodone**—antidepressant
**nifedipine**—antihypertensive
**Nitro-Bid**—antianginal, antihypertensive, coronary vasodilatory
**Nitro-Dur**—antianginal, antihypertensive, coronary vasodilator
**nitroglycerin**—antianginal, antihypertensive, coronary vasodilator
**Nitrostat**—antianginal
**Nolvadex**—antineoplastic, hormonal/biological response
**Norpramin**—antidepressant
**nortriptyline hydrochloride**—antidepressant
**Novolin**—antidiabetic
**Novoprofen**—analgesic
**NPH insulin**—antidiabetic
**Nubain**—analgesic
**Nuprin**—analgesic

**Oretic**—antihypertensive
**Orinase**—antidiabetic

**Pamelor**—antidepressant
**Pamprin-IB**—analgesic
**Panadol**—analgesic
**paroxetine**—antidepressant
**Paxil**—antidepressant
**penicillin V potassium**—penicillin, antibiotic
**Pen-Vee K**—penicillin, antibiotic
**Percocet**—analgesic
**Pertofrane**—antidepressant
**Phenergan**—antiemetic, antitussive, expectorant
**Phenergan with Codeine**—antitussive, expectorant
**phenobarbital**—anticonvulsant, antianxiety, sedative hypnotic
**Phentermine hydrochloride**—anorexiant
**phenytoin**—anticonvulsant
**potassium chloride**—electrolyte, water balance, vitamin, mineral
**prednisone**—corticosteroids, antiarthritic
**primidone**—anticonvulsant
**procainamide**—antiarrhythmic
**Procan SR**—antiarrhythmic
**Procardia**—antihypertensive
**progesterone**—hormone
**promethazine hydrochloride**—antiemetic, antitussive, expectorant
**Pronestyl**—antiarrhythmic

**propoxyphene**—analgesic
**propranolol hydrochloride**—antianginal, antiarrhythmic, antihypertensive, antimigraine, beta blocker
**Protostat**—antibacterial, antiprotozoal
**protriptyline**—antidepressant
**Proventil**—bronchodilator, antiasthmatic
**Proventil Inhaler**—antiasthmatic, bronchodilator
**Provera**—contraceptive, progestin
**Prozac**—antidepressant

**Reglan**—antiemetic, acid/peptic
**Relafen**—NSAID
**Restoril**—sedative hypnotic
**Ritalin**—CNS stimulant
**Ritalin-SR**—CNS stimulant
**Roxanol**—analgesic
**Rufen**—NSAID, antiarthritic, analgesic, antipyretic

**Septra**—sulfonamide, antimicrobial
**sertraline**—antidepressant
**Sinequam**—antidepressant, antianxiety
**Sinequan Concentrate**—antidepressant
**Slo-Bid**—antiasthmatic
**Slo-Phyllin**—antiasthmatic
**Slow-K**—electrolyte, water balance, vitamin, mineral
**Solfoton**—anticonvulsant
**Soma**—skeletal muscle relaxant
**sulfamethoxazole trimethoprim**—sulfonamide, antimicrobial
**Tagamet**—acid/peptic disorder
**tamoxifen citrate**—antineoplastic, hormonal/biological response

**Tegretol**—anticonvulsant
**temazepam**—sedative hypnotic
**Tempra**—analgesic, antipyretic
**Ten-K**—electrolyte, water balance, vitamin, mineral
**Tenormin**—antianginal, antihypertensive, beta blocker
**terbutaline**—bronchodilator
**Tessalon Perles**—antitussant
**Theo-24**—antiasthmatic
**Theo-Dur**—antiasthmatic, bronchodilator
**theophylline**—bronchodilator, antiasthmatic
**Tofranil**—antidepressant
**tolbutamde**—antidiabetic
**T-Phyl**—bronchodilator
**trazodone hydrochloride**—analgesic, antianxiety, antidepressant, antiarthritic
**Triadapin**—antidepressant
**triamcinolone acetonide**—corticosteriod, sulfonamide, antiasthmatic
**trimipramine**—antidepressant
**Trimox**—penicillin, antibiotic
**Tripramine**—antidepressant
**Tylenol**—analgesic, antipyretic
**Tylenol with Codeine**—analgesic
**Tylox**—analgesic

**Uniphyl**—bronchodilator

**Valium**—antianxiety, anticonvulsant, skeletal muscle relaxant
**valproic acid**—anticonvulsant
**V-Cillin K**—penicillin

# Common Prescribed and Over-the-Counter Medications

**Ventolin**—bronchodilator
**verapamil**—antiarrhythmic, antihypertensive
**Verelan**—antiarrhythmic, antianginal, antiarthritic,
    antihypertensive, calcium channel blocker
**Vibramycin**—tetracycline, antibiotic
**Vicodin**—analgesic
**Vivactil**—antidepressant
**Voltaren**—analgesic, antiarthritic, NSAID

**warfarin sodium**—anticoagulant
**Wellbutrin**—antidepressant
**Wymox**—penicillin, antibiotic
**Wytensin**—antihypertensive

**Xanax**—antianxiety, sedative

**Zoloft**—antidepressant
**Zonalon**—antianxiety, antidepressant
**Zovirax**—antiviral
**Zyloprim**—antigout

### ➤ AIDS (ACQUIRED IMMUNE DEFICIENCY SYNDROME)

*Mode of transmission*—infected blood via intravenous drug use, unprotected sexual contact, blood transfusions or (rarely) accidental needle sticks. Mothers also may pass HIV to their unborn children.
*Incubation*—several months or years.

### ➤ CHICKENPOX (VARICELLA)

*Mode of transmission*—airborne droplets. Can also be spread by contact with open sores.
*Incubation*—11 to 21 days.

### ➤ GERMAN MEASLES (RUBELLA)

*Mode of transmission*—airborne droplets. Mothers may pass the disease to unborn children.
*Incubation*—10 to 12 days.

### ➤ VIRAL HEPATITIS

*Mode of transmission*—blood, stool, or other body fluids, or contaminated objects.
*Incubation*—weeks to months, depending on type.

### ➤ MENINGITIS, BACTERIAL

*Mode of transmission*—oral and nasal secretions.
*Incubation*—2 to 10 days.

### ➤ MUMPS

*Mode of transmission*—droplets of saliva or objects
    contaminated by saliva.
*Incubation*—14 to 24 days.

### ➤ PNEUMONIA, BACTERIAL AND VIRAL

*Mode of transmission*—oral and nasal droplets and
    secretions.
*Incubation*—several days.

### ➤ STAPHYLOCOCCAL SKIN INFECTION

*Mode of transmission*—direct contact with infected
    wounds or sores or with contaminated objects.
*Incubation*—several days.

### ➤ TUBERCULOSIS (TB)

*Mode of transmission*—respiratory secretions, air-
    borne, or on contaminated objects.
*Incubation*—2 to 6 weeks.

### ➤ WHOOPING COUGH (PERTUSSIS)

*Mode of transmission*—respiratory secretions or air-
    borne droplets.
*Incubation*—6 to 20 days.

### ➤ AIRBORNE INFECTION

(such as TB)

- You have transported a patient who is infected with a life-threatening airborne disease, but you are not aware that the patient is infected.
- After the medical facility diagnoses the disease in the patient, they must notify your designated officer (DO) within 48 hours.
- Your DO then notifies you that you have been exposed.
- Your employer arranges for you to be evaluated, with a followup by a doctor or appropriate other health care professional.

### ➤ BLOODBORNE INFECTION

(such as HIV or HBV)

- You have come into contact with blood and body fluids of a patient, and you wonder if that patient is infected with a life-threatening disease such as HIV or HBV.
- You seek immediate medical attention and document the incident for worker's compensation.
- You ask your designated officer (DO) to determine if you have been exposed to an infectious disease.
- Your DO must gather information and, if warranted, consults the medical facility to which the patient was transported.
- The medical facility must gather information and report findings to your DO within 48 hours.
- Your DO notifies you of the findings.
- Your employer arranges for you to be evaluated, with a follow up by a doctor or appropriate other health care professional.

| = | equal. |
|---|---|
| + | positive. |
| − | negative. |
| > | greater than. |
| < | less than. |
| × | times or multiply. |
| @ | at. |
| Δ | change. |
| a̅ | before. |
| **AAA** | abdominal aortic aneurysm. |
| **AAL** | anterior axillary line. |
| **ABCs** | airway, breathing, circulation. |
| **Abd** | abdominal. |
| **ADD** | attention deficit disorder. |
| **ADHD** | attention deficit hyperactivity disorder. |
| **AED** | automated external defibrillator. |
| **AIDS** | acquired immune deficiency syndrome. |
| **ALS** | advanced life support. |
| **AMA** | against medical advice. |
| **AMI** | acute myocardial infarction. |
| **AMS** | altered mental status. |
| **A/O** | alert and oriented. |
| **A/P** | anterior and posterior. |
| **APE** | acute pulmonary edema. |
| **APGAR** | appearance, pulse, grimace, activity, respiratory effort. |
| **ASHD** | arteriosclerotic heart disease. |
| **ATV** | automatic transport ventilator. |
| **AVPU** | alert, verbally responsive, painful response, unresponsive. |

| | |
|---|---|
| **BAC** | blood alcohol content. |
| **BG** | blood glucose. |
| **b.i.d.** | twice daily. |
| **BLS** | basic life support. |
| **b.m.** | bowel movement. |
| **BP** | blood pressure. |
| **bpm** | beats per minute. |
| **BSA** | body surface area. |
| **BSI** | body substance isolation. |
| **BVM** | bag-valve-mask resuscitator. |
| **c̄** | with. |
| **CABG** | coronary artery bypass graft. |
| **CAD** | coronary artery disease. |
| **c/c** | chief complaint. |
| **cc** | cubic centimeter. |
| **CCU** | critical care unit. |
| **CHF** | congestive heart failure. |
| **CISM** | critical incident stress management. |
| **CNS** | central nervous system. |
| **c/o** | complained of. |
| **CO** | carbon monoxide. |
| **CO$_2$** | carbon dioxide. |
| **COPD** | chronic obstructive pulmonary disease. |
| **CPR** | cardiopulmonary resuscitation. |
| **CSF** | cerebrospinal fluid. |
| **CT** | computerized tomography. |
| **CUPS** | critical, unstable, potentially unstable, stable. |
| **CVA** | cerebrovascular accident. |

| | |
|---|---|
| **D5W** | 5 percent dextrose in water. |
| **DAN** | Diver's Alert Network. |
| **d/c** | discontinue. |
| **DKA** | diabetic ketoacidosis. |
| **DNAR** | do not attempt resuscitation. |
| **DNR** | do not resuscitate. |
| **DOA** | dead on arrival. |
| **DOB** | date of birth. |
| **Dr.** | doctor. |
| **DTs** | delirium tremens. |
| **Dx** | diagnosis. |
| | |
| **ECG** | electrocardiogram. Also called EKG. |
| **ED** | emergency department. |
| **EEG** | electroencephalogram. |
| **EENT** | ears, eyes, nose, throat. |
| **EID** | esophageal intubation device. |
| **EMD** | emergency medical dispatch. |
| **EMS** | emergency medical services. |
| **EMT** | emergency medical technician. |
| **EMT-B** | EMT-Basic. |
| **EMT-I** | EMT-Intermediate. |
| **EMT-P** | EMT-Paramedic. |
| **EOA** | esophageal obturator airway. |
| **EPI** | epinephrine. |
| **ER** | emergency room. |
| **ET** | endotracheal tube. |
| **ETA** | estimated time of arrival. |
| **EtCO$_2$** | end-tidal carbon dioxide. |
| **EtOH** | ethyl alcohol. |

| | |
|---|---|
| **FBAO** | foreign body airway obstruction |
| **FROPVD** | flow-restricted oxygen-powered ventilation device. |
| **FUO** | fever of unknown origin. |
| **fx** | fracture. |
| | |
| **GCS** | Glasgow Coma Score. |
| **GI** | gastrointestinal. |
| **GSW** | gunshot wound. |
| **gtt** | drops. |
| **GU** | genitourinary. |
| **GYN** | gynecology. |
| | |
| **H** | hour. |
| **HBV** | hepatitis B virus. |
| **HIV** | human immunodeficiency virus. |
| | |
| **Hx** | history. |
| | |
| **ICP** | intracranial pressure. |
| **ICS** | incident command system. |
| **ICU** | intensive care unit. |
| **IM** | intramuscular. |
| **IMS** | incident management system. |
| **IO** | intraosseous. |
| **IUD** | intrauterine device. |
| **IV** | intravenous. |
| **IVP** | intravenous push. |
| | |
| **JVD** | jugular vein distention. |

| | |
|---|---|
| **KED** | Kendrick Extrication Device. |
| **kg** | kilogram. |
| **KVO** | keep vein open. |
| | |
| **l** | liter. |
| **L.** | left |
| **LLQ** | left lower quadrant (of abdomen). |
| **LPN** | licensed practical nurse. |
| **LOC** | loss of or level of consciousness. |
| **LR** | lactated ringer's. |
| **LUQ** | left upper quadrant (of abdomen). |
| | |
| **MAST** | military anti-shock trousers. |
| **MCI** | multiple-casualty incident. |
| **MD** | physician. |
| **mg** | milligram. |
| **MI** | myocardial infarction. |
| **ml** | milliliter. |
| **mm** | millimeter. |
| **mm Hg** | millimeters mercury. |
| **MOI** | mechanism of injury. |
| **MPDS** | medical priority dispatch system. |
| **MRI** | magnetic resonance imaging. |
| **MS-ABC** | mental status, airway, breathing, circulation. |
| **MVA** | motor-vehicle accident. |
| **MVC** | motor vehicle crash. |
| | |
| **N/A** | not applicable. |
| **NG** | nasogastric. |
| **NKA** | no known allergies. |
| **NKDA** | no known drug allergies. |

| | |
|---|---|
| **NPA** | nasopharyngeal (nasal) airway. |
| **NRB** | nonrebreather face mask. |
| **NS** | normal saline. |
| **NSR** | normal sinus rhythm. |
| **NTG** | nitroglycerin. |
| **N/V** | nausea and vomiting. |
| | |
| **O₂** | oxygen. |
| **OB/GYN** | obstetrics and gynecology. |
| **OD** | overdose. |
| **OPA** | oropharyngeal (oral) airway. |
| **OPQRST** | onset, provocation, quality, referral, radiation, region, severity, time. |
| **OR** | operating room. |
| **O.T.C.** | over the counter. |
| **oz.** | ounce. |
| | |
| **P** | pulse. |
| **P.A.** | physician assistant. |
| **PASG** | pneumatic anti-shock garment. |
| **PCR** | prehospital care report. |
| **PE** | physical exam. |
| **PEA** | pulseless electrical activity. |
| **PEARL** | pupils equal and reactive to light. |
| **PIAA** | personal injury auto accident. |
| **PID** | pelvic inflammatory disease. |
| **PMH** | past medical history. |
| **PMS** | pulses, motor ability, and sensory response; premenstrual syndrome. |
| **PPE** | personal protective equipment. |
| **p.o.** | by mouth. |

| | |
|---|---|
| **p.r.n.** | as needed. |
| **p.s.i.** | pounds per square inch. |
| **PSAP** | public safety access point. |
| **pt** | patient; pint. |
| **q.** | every. |
| **q.d.** | every day. |
| **q.h.** | every hour. |
| **q.i.d.** | four times a day. |
| **qod** | every other day. |
| | |
| **R.** | right. |
| **RBC** | red blood cells. |
| **RLQ** | right lower quadrant (of abdomen). |
| **RMA** | refused medical assistance. |
| **RN** | registered nurse. |
| **r/o** | rule out. |
| **R.O.M.** | range of motion. |
| **RR** | respiratory rate. |
| **RUQ** | right upper quadrant (of abdomen). |
| **R$_x$** | prescription. |
| | |
| **$\overline{s}$** | without. |
| **SA** | sinoatrial. |
| **SAMPLE** | symptoms, allergies, meds, pertinent past medical hx, last oral intake, events leading up to. |
| **s.c.** | subcutaneous. Also called sq. |
| **SIDS** | sudden infant death syndrome. |
| **SL** | sublingual. |
| **SOB** | shortness of breath. |
| **sq.** | subcutaneous. Also called s.c. |

| | |
|---|---|
| **S.T.D.** | sexually transmitted disease. |
| **START** | simple triage and rapid transport. |
| | |
| **TB** | tuberculosis. |
| **TIA** | transient ischemic attack. |
| **t.i.d.** | three times a day. |
| **TKO** | to keep open. |
| **TOT** | turned over to. |
| | |
| **URI** | upper respiratory infection. |
| **UTI** | urinary tract infection. |
| **VD** | venereal disease. |
| **V.S.** | vital signs. |
| **VF** | ventricular fibrillation. |
| | |
| **w/** | with. |
| **WBC** | white blood cells. |
| **WNL** | within normal limits. |
| **w/o** | without. |
| | |
| **y/o** | year old. |

**abduction**   movement away from the body's midline.
**adduction**   movement toward the body's midline.
**afferent**   conducting toward a structure.
**anatomical position**   body is erect with arms down at
     sides, palms front.
**anterior**   the front surface of the body.
**anterior to**   in front of.

**caudad**   toward the tail.
**cephalad**   toward the head.
**circumduction**   circular movement of a part.
**coronal plane**   an imaginary plane that passes
     through body from side to side and divides it into
     front and back sections. Also called frontal plane.
**craniad**   toward the cranium.

**deep**   situated remote from surface.
**distal**   situated away from point of origin.
**dorsal**   pertaining to the back surface of body.
**dorsiflexion**   bending backward.

**efferent**   conducting away from a structure.
**elevation**   raising a body part.
**extension**   stretching or moving jointed parts into or
     toward a straight condition.
**external**   situated outside.

**flexion**   bending or moving jointed parts closer
     together.
**frontal plane**   an imaginary plane that passes through
     body from side to side and divides it into front and
     back sections. Also called coronal plane.

**inferior**   situated below.
**internal**   situated inside.

**lateral**   situated away from the body's midline.
**lateral rotation**   rotating outward away from the
body's midline.
**left lateral recumbent**   lying down or reclining on
left side.
**mediad**   toward the midline of body.
**medial**   situated toward body's midline.
**medial rotation**   rotating inward toward body's midline.
**midsagittal plane**   an imaginary plane that passes
through body from front to back and divides it into
right and left halves.

**palmar**   concerning inner surface of hand.
**peripheral**   away from a central structure.
**plantar**   concerning the sole of the foot.
**posterior**   pertaining to back surface of body.
**posterior to**   situated behind.
**pronation**   lying face downward or turning hand so
palm faces downward or backward.
**prone**   lying face down and flat.
**protraction**   a pushing forward of part of body, such
as mandible.
**proximal**   situated nearest the point of origin.

**recumbent**   lying down, reclining.
**retraction a drawing back, as of the tongue.**
**right lateral recumbent**   lying down on right side.

**rotation**   turning around an axis.

**sagittal plane**   an imaginary plane parallel to medial
  plane; passes through body from front to back and
  divides body into right and left sections.
**superficial**   situated near surface.
**superior**   situated above.
**supination**   lying face upward or turning hand so
  palm faces forward or upward.
**supine**   lying down flat on back and face up.

**transverse plane**   an imaginary plane that passes
  through body and divides it into upper and lower
  sections.

**ventral**   front surface of body.

Prefixes are followed by a dash. Suffixes are preceded by a dash. All others are combining forms, which usually have a slash and a vowel following the word root.

**a-**  not, without, lacking, deficient.
**ab-**  away from.
**-able**  capable of.
**abdomin/o**  abdomen.
**ac-**  to, toward, pertaining to.
**acou**  hear.
**acr/o**  extremity, top, peak.
**acu-**  with a needle.
**ad-**  to, toward.
**aden/o**  gland.
**adip/o**  fat.
**-aemia**  blood.
**aer/o**  air.
**-aesthesia**  sensation.
**-algesia**  painful.
**-algia**  painful.
**af-**  to.
**algi-**  pain.
**all-**  other.
**ambi-**  both sides.
**ambly/o**  dim, dull, lazy.
**amph-**  on both sides, around both.
**amyl/o**  starch.
**an-**  without, negative.
**ana-**  upward, again, backward, excess.
**andr/o**  man, male.
**angi/o**  blood vessel, duct.

**anis/o**   unequal.
**ankyl/o**   stiff.
**ant-**   against, opposed to, preventing.
**ante-**   before, in front of.
**antero-**   from front to.
**anti-**   against, opposed to, preventing.
**ap-**   to.
**apo-**   separation, derivation from.
**-arium**   place for something.
**arteri/o**   artery.
**arthr/o**   joint, articulation.
**articul/o**   joint.
**as-**   to.
**-ase**   enzyme.
**at-**   to.
**audi/o**   hearing.
**aur/o**   ear.
**aut/o**   self.

**bi-**   two, twice, double, both.
**bis-**   twice, double.
**bi/o**   life.
**blephar/o**   eyelid.
**brachi/o**   upper arm.
**brady-**   slow.
**bronch/o**   larger air passages of lungs.
**bucc/o**   cheek.

**cac/o**   bad, evil.
**calc/o**   stone.
**calcane/o**   heel.

**calor/o**   heat.
**cancr/o**   cancer.
**capit/o**   head.
**caps/o**   container.
**carcin/o**   cancer.
**cardi/o**   heart.
**carp/o**   wrist bone.
**cat-**   down, lower, under, against, along with.
**cata-**   down, lower, under, against, along with.
**-cele**   tumor, a cyst, hernia.
**celi/o**   abdomen.
**cent**   hundred.
**-centesis**   perforation, puncture, or tapping with a needle.
**cephal/o**   head.
**cerebr/o**   cerebrum.
**cervic/o**   neck, cervix.
**cheil/o**   lip.
**cheir/o**   hand.
**chil/o**   lip.
**chir/o**   hand.
**chlor/o**   green.
**chol/e**   bile, gall.
**chondr/o**   cartilage.
**chrom/o**   color.
**chromat/o**   color.
**chron/o**   time.
**-cid**   cut, kill, fall.
**-cide**   causing death.
**circum-**   around.
**-cis**   cut, kill, fall.

**clysis**   irrigation.
**co-**   with.
**col-**   with.
**col/o**   colon, large intestine.
**colp/o**   vagina.
**com-**   with, together.
**con-**   together.
**contra-**   against, opposite.
**cor/e**   pupil.
**cost/o**   rib.
**crani/o**   skull.
**cry/o**   cold.
**crypt/o**   hide, cover, conceal.
**cyan/o**   blue.
**cyst/o**   urinary bladder, cyst, sac of fluid.
**-cyte**   cell.
**cyt/o**   cell.

**dacry/o**   tear.
**dactyl/o**   finger, toe.
**de-**   down, from, not.
**deca-**   ten.
**deci-**   tenth.
**demi-**   half.
**dent/o**   tooth.
**derm/o**   skin.
**dermat/o**   skin.
**dextr/o**   right.
**di-**   twice, double.
**dia-**   through, across, apart.
**dipl/o**   double, twin, twice.

**dips/o**   thirst.
**dis-**   to free, to undo.
**dors/o**   back.
**-dynia**   pain.
**dys-**   bad, difficult, abnormal, incomplete.

**-ectasia**   dilation or enlargement of organ or part.
**ecto-**   outer, outside of.
**-ectomy**   the surgical removal of organ/part.
**ef-**   out.
**electr/o**   electric.
**emesis**   vomiting.
**-emia**   condition of the blood.
**en-**   in, into, within.
**encephal/o**   brain.
**end-**   within.
**endo-**   within.
**ent-**   within, inner.
**ento-**   within, inner.
**enter/o**   small intestine.
**ep-**   over, on, upon.
**epi-**   over, on, upon.
**erythr/o**   red.
**-esthesia**   feeling, sensation.
**eu-**   good, well, normal, healthy.
**ex-**   out of, away from.
**exo-**   outside, outward.
**extra-**   on the outside, beyond, in addition to.

**faci/o**   face, surface.
**febr/i**   fever.

**-ferent**   bear, carry.
**fibr/o**   fiber, filament.
**fore-**   before, in front of.
**-form**   shape.
**-fugal**   moving away, passing from.
**-fuge**   one that drives away.

**galact/o**   milk.
**gangli/o**   mass, knot.
**-gaster**   stomach, belly.
**gastr/o**   stomach.
**gen/o**   come into being, originate.
**-genesis**   production or origin.
**-genic**   giving rise to, originating in.
**gloss/o**   tongue.
**glyc/o**   sweet.
**gnath/o**   jaw.
**gnos/o**   knowledge.
**-gog**   to make flow.
**-gogue**   to make flow.
**-gram**   drawing, written record.
**-graph**   an instrument for recording activity of an
   organ.
**-graphy**   the recording of the activity of an organ.
**gynec/o**   woman.

**hem/a**   blood.
**hem/o**   blood.
**hemat/o**   blood.
**hemi-**   one-half.
**hepat/o**   liver.

**heter/o**   other, dissimilarity.
**hidr/o**   sweat.
**hist/o**   tissue.
**hol/o**   all, entire, total, complete.
**hom/o**   same, similar, unchanging constant.
**home/o**   same, similar, unchanging constant.
**hyal/o**   glass.
**hydr/o**   water, fluid.
**hyp-**   under.
**hyper-**   beyond, normal, excessive.
**hypn/o**   sleep.
**hypo-**   below normal, deficient, under, beneath.
**hyster/o**   uterus, womb.

**-iasis**   condition, pathological state.
**iatr/o**   healer, physician.
**-ible**   capable of.
**-id**   in a state, condition of.
**idio-**   peculiar, separate, distinct.
**il-**   negative, prefix.
**ile/o**   ileum.
**ili/o**   ilium.
**im-**   negative, prefix.
**in-**   in, into, within.
**infra-**   beneath, below.
**inter-**   between.
**intra-**   within.
**intro-**   within, into.
**irid/o**   iris.
**ischi/o**   ischium.
**-ism**   condition, theory.

**-ismus**   abnormal condition.
**iso-**   same, equal, alike.
**-itis**   inflammation.
**-ize**   to treat by special method.

**juxta**   near, nearby.

**karyo**   nucleus, nut.
**kata-**   down, against.
**kera-**   horn, indicates hardness.
**kerat/o**   cornea.
**kinesi/o**   movement, motion.
**-kinesis**   motion.

**labi/o**   lip.
**lact/o**   milk.
**lal/o**   talk.
**lapar/o**   flank, abdomen, abdominal wall.
**laryng/o**   larynx.
**later/o**   side.
**lept/o**   thin, small, soft.
**leuc/o**   white.
**leuk/o**   white.
**lingu/o**   tongue.
**lip/o**   fat.
**lith/o**   stone.
**-logist**   a person who studies.
**log/o**   speak.
**-logy**   study of.
**lumb/o**   loin.
**lymph/o**   lymph.

**-lysis**   destruction.

**macr/o**   large, long.
**mal-**   bad, poor, evil.
**malac/o**   a softening.
**mamm/o**   breast.
**-mania**   mental aberration.
**mast/o**   breast.
**medi/o**   middle.
**mega-**   large.
**megal/o**   large.
**-megaly**   an enlargement.
**melan/o**   dark, black.
**men/o**   month.
**mes/o**   middle.
**meta-**   change, transformation, exchange.
**-meter**   measure.
**metr/o**   uterus.
**micr/o**   small.
**mi/o**   less, smaller.
**mon/o**   single, only, sole.
**morph/o**   form.
**multi-**   many, much.
**myc/o**   fungus.
**mycet/o**   fungus.
**my/o**   muscle.
**myel/o**   marrow, also refers to spinal cord.
**myx/o**   mucus, slimelike.

**narc/o**   stupor, numbness.
**nas/o**   nose.

**ne/o**  new.
**necr/o**  corpse.
**nephr/o**  kidney.
**neur/o**  nerve.
**niter-**  nitrogen.
**nitro-**  nitrogen.
**noct/i**  night.
**non-**  not.
**norm/o**  rule, order, normal.
**nucleo-**  nucleus.
**null/i**  none.
**nyct/o**  night.

**ob-**  against, in front of, toward.
**ocul/o**  eye.
**odont/o**  tooth.
**-oid**  shape, form, resemblance.
**olig/o**  few, deficient, scanty.
**-oma**  tumor, swelling.
**omo-**  shoulder.
**o/o-**  egg.
**onych/o**  nail.
**oophor/o**  ovary.
**opisth-**  backward.
**-opsy**  a viewing.
**opthalm/o**  eye.
**opt/o**  sight, vision.
**optic/o**  sight, vision.
**or/o**  mouth.
**orch/o**  testicle.
**orchid/o**  testicle.

**-orium**   place for something.
**orth/o**   straight, upright.
**os-**   mouth, bone.
**-osis**   process, an abnormal condition.
**oste/o**   bone.
**-ostomosis**   to furnish with a mouth or outlet.
**-otomy**   cutting.
**ot/o**   ear.
**ovari/o**   ovary.
**ov/i**   egg.
**ov/o**   egg.
**oxy-**   sharp, acid.

**pachy-**   thicken.
**palat/o**   palate.
**pan-**   all entire, every.
**para-**   beside, beyond, accessory to, apart from,
     against.
**path/o**   disease.
**-pathy**   disease of a part.
**-penia**   an abnormal reduction.
**peps/o**   digestion.
**pept/o**   digestion.
**per-**   throughout, completely, extremely.
**peri-**   around, surrounding.
**-pexy**   fixation.
**phag/o**   ear.
**pharyng/o**   throat.
**phas/o**   speech.
**phil/o**   like, have an affinity for.
**phleb/o**   vein.

**-phobia**   fear, dread.
**phon/o**   sound.
**phor/o**   bear, carry.
**phot/o**   light.
**phren/o**   diaphragm.
**-phylaxis**   protection.
**physi/o**   nature.
**pil/o**   hair.
**-plasia**   development, formation.
**-plasm**   to mold.
**-plasty**   surgical repair.
**-plegia**   paralysis, a stroke.
**pleur/o**   rib, side, pleura.
**plur**   more.
**pnea-**   breath, breathing.
**pneum/o**   lung, air, breath.
**pneumat/o**   air, breath.
**pneumon/o**   lung.
**pod/o**   foot.
**-poies**   is formation.
**poly-**   much, many.
**post-**   after, behind.
**pre-**   before.
**pro-**   before, in front of.
**proto**   first.
**proct/o**   anus.
**pseud/o**   false.
**psych/o**   mind, soul.
**-ptosis**   abnormal dropping/sagging of part.
**pulmon/o**   lung.
**py/o**   pus.

**pyel/o**   renal pelvis.
**pyr/o**   fire, fever.

**quadri-**   four.

**rach/i**   spine.
**radio-**   ray, radiation.
**re-**   back, against, contrary.
**rect/o**   rectum.
**ren/o**   kidneys.
**retro-**   located behind, backward.
**-rhage**   hemorrhage, flow.
**-rhaphy**   a suturing or stitching.
**-rhea**   to flow, indicates discharge.
**rhin/o**   nose.
**-rrhage**   abnormal discharge.
**-rrhagia**   hemorrhage from organ/body part.
**-rrhea**   flowing or discharge.

**sacchar**   sugar.
**sacr/o**   sacrum.
**salping-**   a tube, relating to a fallopian tube.
**sanguin/o**   blood.
**sarc/o**   flesh.
**schiz/o**   split.
**scler/o**   hardening.
**-sclerosis**   hardening condition.
**scoli/o**   twisted, crooked.
**-scope**   an instrument for observing.
**-scopy**   to see.
**-sect**   cut.

**semi-**   one-half, partly.
**seps/o**   infection.
**sept/o**   infection.
**somat/o**   body.
**son/o**   sound.
**spermat/o**   sperm, semen.
**sphygm/o**   pulse.
**splen/o**   spleen.
**-stasis**   stopping, controlling.
**sten/o**   narrow.
**stere/o**   solid, three-dimensional.
**steth/o**   chest.
**sthen/o**   strength.
**-stomy**   surgically creating a new opening.
**sub-**   under, near, almost, moderately.
**super-**   above, excess.
**supra-**   above, over.
**sym-**   joined together, with.
**syn-**   joined together, with.

**tachy-**   fast.
**tele-**   distant, far.
**tetra-**   four.
**therm/o**   heat.
**thio-**   sulfur.
**thorac/o**   chest cavity.
**thromb/o**   clot, lump.
**thyro-**   thyroid gland.
**-tome**   surgical instrument for cutting.
**-tomy**   surgical operation on organ/body part.
**top/o**   place.

**trache/o**   trachea.
**trans-**   through, across, beyond.
**tri-**   three.
**trich/o**   hair.
**-tripsy**   surgical crushing.
**troph/o**   nourish.

**ultra-**   beyond, excess.
**uni-**   one.
**ur/o**   urine.
**ureter/o**   ureter.
**urethr/o**   urethra.
**-uria**   relating to urine.

**vas/o**   vessel, duct.
**ven/o**   vein.
**ventr/o**   belly, cavity.
**vesic/o**   blister, bladder.
**viscer/o**   internal organ.

**xanth/o**   yellow.
**xen/o**   stranger.
**xer/o**   dry.

**zo/o**   animal life.

## Ambulance-to-Hospital Radio Report

- Unit identification (Ambulance # _____)
- Level of provider. _____
- Estimated time of arrival (ETA). _____
- Patient's age and sex. _____
- Chief complaint (why the patient called ambulance). _____
- Brief, pertinent history of present illness or injury. _____
- Major past illnesses. _____
- Mental status (AVPU). _____
- Baseline vital signs. _____
- Pertinent findings of physical exam. _____
- Emergency medical care given. _____
- Response to emergency medical care. _____
- Does medical direction have any questions or orders? _____

*NOTE: There are a number of local formats for radio reports, which may differ somewhat from the example above. However, they all adhere to the same basic principles. They should follow a logical order, be concise, and paint a picture of patient's problem and priorities for hospital care.

## This Pocket Reference Belongs to:

_____

**Important Phone Numbers**

911 Dispatch Center _____

American Red Cross _____

CHEMTREC Emergency 1-800-424-9300

CHEMTREC Non-emergency 1-800-262-8200

CISD Team _____

Child Abuse Hotline_____

Confined Space Rescue _____

Diver's Alert Network _____

HAZMAT Team _____

High-Angle Rescue _____

Hospital _____

Hospital _____

Hospital _____

Hospital _____

Medical Examiner / Coroner _____

Poison Control Center _____

Water Rescue Team _____